HERBAL

PLANT

IDENTIFICATION

BOOK

Explore the Healing Power in Natural Medicinal Plants for Common Ailments to Improve your Wellness Including Health Benefits and More

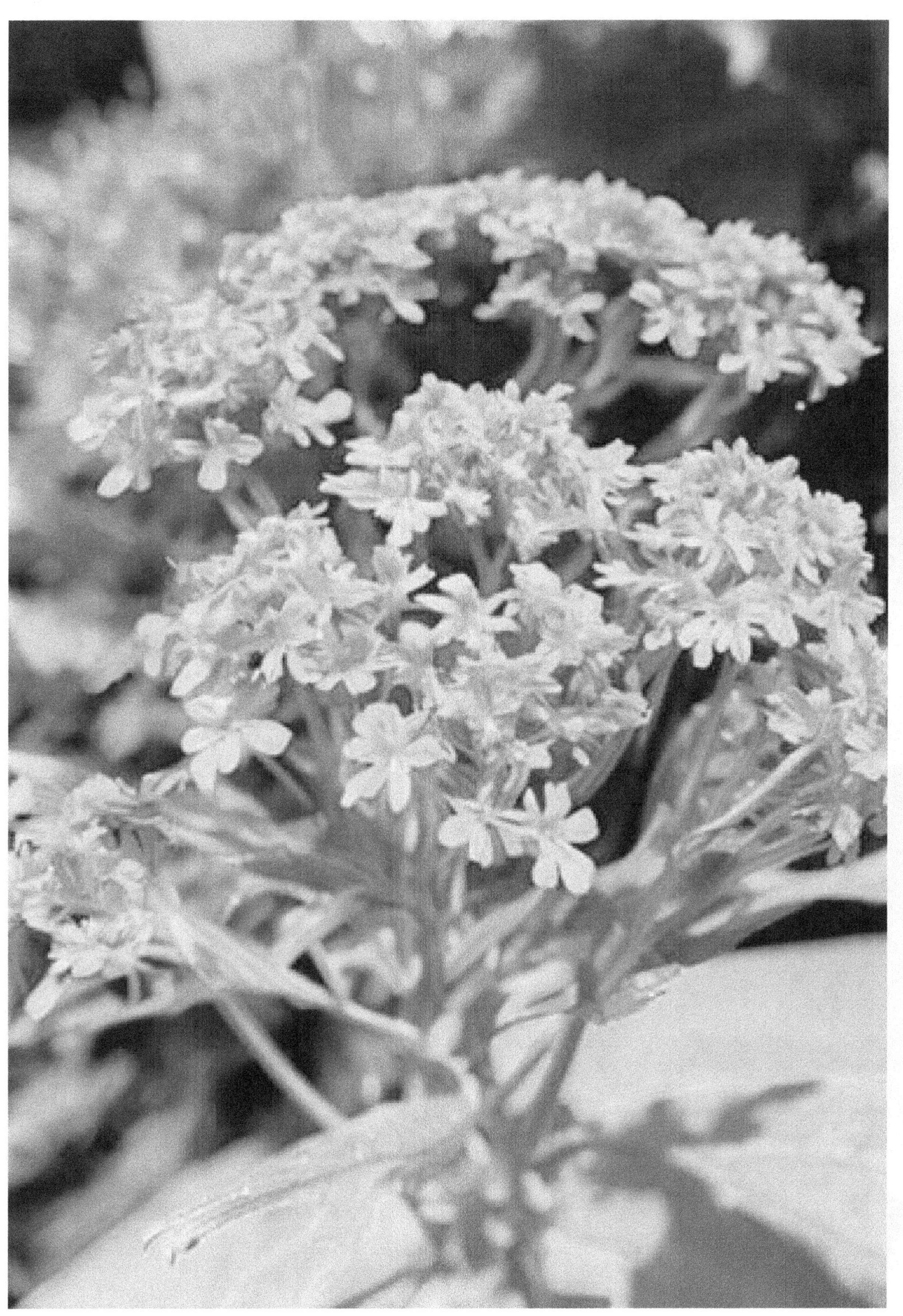

Copyright: © 2024 by Dr. Gary C. Wong

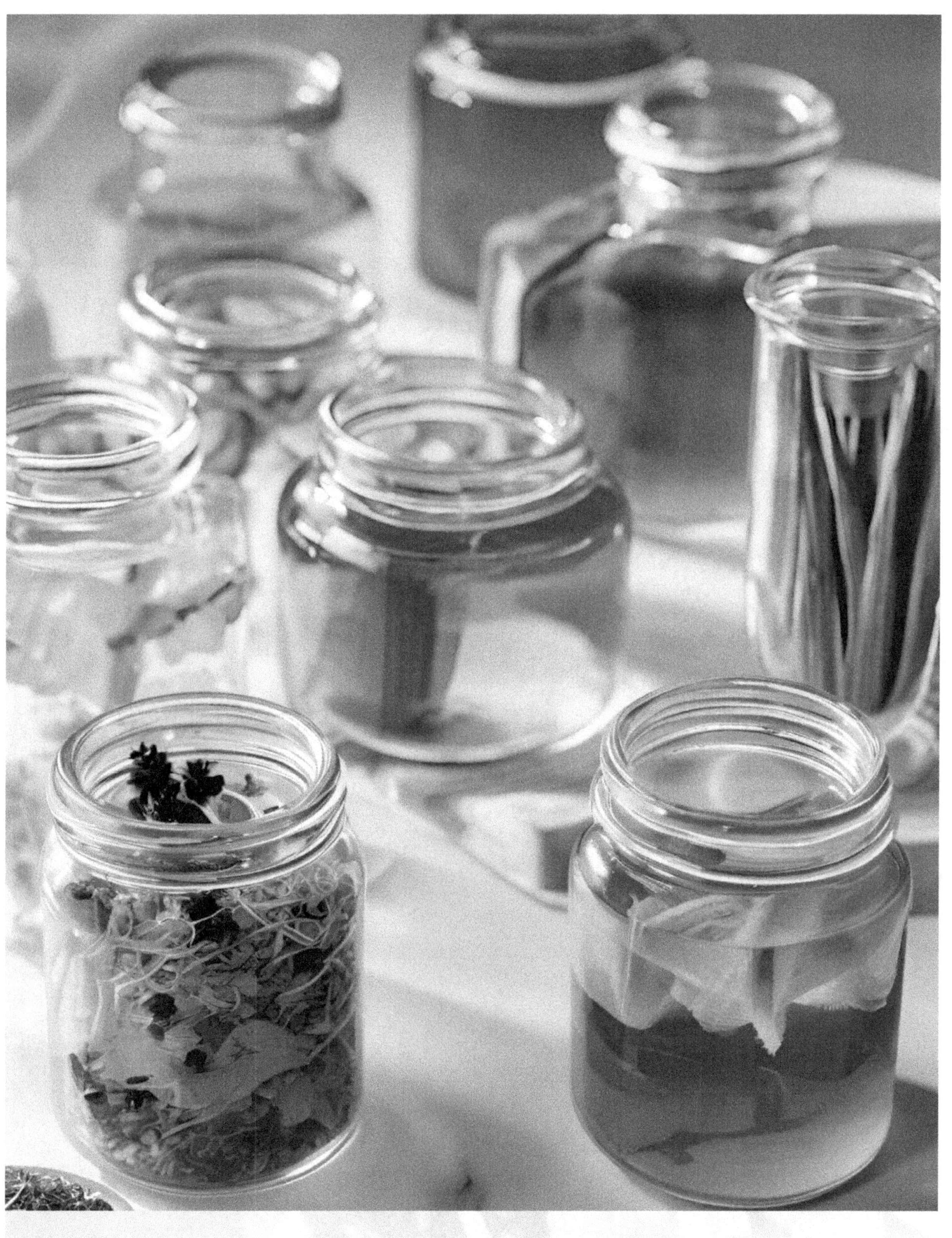

TABLE OF CONTENT

INTRODUCTION

Herbal plants are nature's pharmacy, a rich repository of therapeutic agents and healing compounds. They are plants that possess medicinal properties, used for their flavor, scent, or therapeutic attributes. These plants, encompassing a wide range of species from different botanical families, have been harnessed by humans for thousands of years. The term "herbal" typically refers to the leafy green parts of the plant, but in the broader context of herbal medicine, it can include roots, seeds, flowers, bark, and berries.

At their core, herbal plants are the living testament to the intricate relationship between humans and nature. They provide us with remedies that are often gentler and more harmonious with our bodies compared to synthetic pharmaceuticals. Each plant has its unique composition of active ingredients, such as alkaloids, glycosides, terpenoids, and flavonoids, which interact with our biological systems to promote health and healing.

The allure of herbal plants lies not only in their medicinal properties but also in their accessibility. Many of these plants can be found in our backyards, gardens, or local forests, waiting to be discovered and utilized. This accessibility empowers individuals to take charge of their health through natural means, fostering a sense of self-reliance and connection to the earth.

Historical Significance of Herbal Plants

The use of herbal plants dates back to the dawn of human civilization. Ancient texts and archaeological findings reveal that early humans utilized plants for healing long before the advent of written language. In ancient Mesopotamia, clay tablets from as early as 3000 BCE list hundreds of medicinal plants, including thyme, myrrh, and opium poppies.

In ancient Egypt, herbal medicine was highly advanced. The Ebers Papyrus, one of the oldest medical documents, written around 1550 BCE, lists over 700 herbal remedies. The Egyptians used garlic for its antibacterial properties, aloe for skin ailments, and castor oil for digestive issues. These practices were not isolated but influenced by trade and interaction with other cultures, spreading knowledge across continents.

The Greeks and Romans further advanced herbal medicine, with figures like Hippocrates and Galen laying the foundations of Western medicine. Hippocrates, often called the "Father of Medicine," emphasized the importance of diet and lifestyle in health, advocating the use of herbs like willow bark (the precursor to aspirin) for pain relief. Galen's extensive writings on herbal medicine shaped medical practice for centuries.

In the East, traditional Chinese medicine (TCM) and Ayurveda in India developed sophisticated systems of herbal medicine. TCM, with its holistic approach, utilizes herbs to balance the body's energies, promoting harmony and health. Ginseng, ginger, and licorice are some of the key herbs in this tradition. Ayurveda, one of the world's oldest holistic healing systems, uses herbs like turmeric, ashwagandha, and neem to treat a variety of ailments and maintain balance between the body, mind, and spirit.

The Middle Ages in Europe saw the rise of herbalism within monasteries, where monks meticulously copied ancient texts and cultivated medicinal gardens. Hildegard of Bingen, a 12th-century abbess, and herbalist, wrote extensively on the healing properties of plants, blending spirituality with medicine. The Renaissance brought a renewed interest in botanical studies, with herbalists like Nicholas Culpeper making herbal knowledge accessible to the common people through his detailed and widely read herbal compendium.

Cultural Uses and Traditions

Herbal plants are deeply woven into the cultural fabric of societies around the world. Each culture has its unique set of beliefs, traditions, and practices surrounding the use of herbs, reflecting the diverse ways in which humans have sought to harness nature's bounty for health and well-being.

In Indigenous cultures, herbal knowledge is often passed down through generations via oral traditions. Native American tribes, for example, use plants like echinacea and sage in their healing rituals and ceremonies. These practices are not merely about physical healing but are intertwined with spiritual beliefs and the connection to the land. The use of herbal smoke, such as burning sage for purification, is a testament to the holistic approach to health that includes the mind, body, and spirit.

In the African continent, traditional healers, known as Sangomas or herbalists, play a crucial role in communities. They use a wide range of plants for healing purposes, often combined with spiritual practices. Plants like African potato and devil's claw are renowned for their medicinal properties. These healers hold vast knowledge of their local flora and are often the first point of contact for health issues within their communities.

Asian cultures have a rich history of herbal medicine that is still very much alive today. In China, traditional medicine shops brimming with dried herbs, roots, and animal parts are a common sight. Traditional Chinese Medicine (TCM) practitioners use these herbs to create personalized remedies based on individual diagnoses. In Japan, Kampo medicine, derived from TCM, integrates herbal treatments with modern medical practices.

In India, Ayurveda remains a vibrant tradition, with millions of people relying on herbal formulations for daily health and chronic conditions. Herbs like holy basil (tulsi), amla (Indian gooseberry), and Brahmi are integral to Ayurvedic practices. Yoga and Ayurveda often go hand in hand, emphasizing the balance of physical, mental, and spiritual health.

European herbal traditions have also evolved over centuries. In the British Isles, the use of herbs is deeply rooted in folklore and local customs. Plants like nettle, elderberry, and chamomile are staples in British herbalism. The Mediterranean region, with its rich biodiversity, boasts a tradition of using herbs like rosemary, oregano, and lavender for both culinary and medicinal purposes.

In the Americas, the blending of Indigenous knowledge with that of European settlers created a unique herbal tradition. The early settlers learned from Native American tribes and incorporated their knowledge into their own practices. The use of herbs like black cohosh, goldenseal, and sassafras became common in early American herbal medicine.

Modern herbalism continues to draw from these ancient traditions while integrating contemporary scientific research. Today, the global resurgence in the interest in natural and holistic health has brought herbal medicine back into the spotlight. People are increasingly turning to herbal remedies as they seek safer, more natural alternatives to synthetic drugs.

Importance of Herbal Plants in Modern Medicine

In an era dominated by rapid scientific advancements and synthetic pharmaceuticals, the importance of herbal plants in modern medicine often remains underestimated. Yet, these natural remedies continue to play a vital role in healthcare systems worldwide. They offer a sustainable, accessible, and often more harmonious approach to healing, addressing the root causes of ailments rather than merely alleviating symptoms.

One of the most compelling reasons for the continued use of herbal plants in modern medicine is their holistic nature. Unlike synthetic drugs, which typically focus on single active ingredients, herbal plants contain a complex mixture of compounds that work synergistically. This complexity can enhance their efficacy and reduce side effects, offering a more balanced and comprehensive approach to treatment. For instance, turmeric, with its active component curcumin, has shown significant anti-inflammatory and antioxidant properties. However, the whole turmeric root, with its blend of curcuminoids and essential oils, often provides more substantial benefits than isolated curcumin alone.

Herbal plants also serve as the foundation for numerous conventional medicines. Aspirin, one of the most widely used drugs globally, originated from salicin found in willow bark. Similarly, the potent anti-malarial drug artemisinin is derived from sweet wormwood (Artemisia annua). These examples underscore the invaluable contributions of herbal plants to the pharmaceutical industry and highlight the potential for discovering new medicines from the plant kingdom.

Moreover, herbal plants align with the growing trend towards personalized medicine. Traditional systems like Ayurveda and Traditional Chinese Medicine (TCM) emphasize tailoring treatments to the individual's constitution and specific needs, a concept now gaining traction in modern healthcare. Herbalists often create customized blends, considering factors such as a person's lifestyle, environment, and overall health, thus providing more targeted and effective treatments.

In addition to their therapeutic properties, herbal plants play a crucial role in preventive medicine. They are rich in antioxidants, vitamins, and minerals that support overall health and strengthen the immune system. Adaptogens like ashwagandha and rhodiola help the body adapt to stress, promoting resilience and preventing illness. As the global population ages and chronic diseases become more prevalent, the preventative and supportive roles of herbal plants are more critical than ever.

Furthermore, the resurgence of interest in natural and holistic health has led to increased scientific research into herbal medicine. Studies on herbs like ginger, garlic, and echinacea have provided robust evidence supporting their use for various conditions. This research not only validates traditional knowledge but also paves the way for integrating herbal medicine into mainstream healthcare.

Herbal plants also offer a sustainable alternative in an age of environmental concerns. Many synthetic drugs are derived from non-renewable resources and involve environmentally damaging processes. In contrast, cultivating and harvesting herbal plants can be done sustainably, supporting biodiversity and reducing the ecological footprint of medicine production.

Overview of the Book Structure

This book is designed to be a comprehensive and accessible guide for anyone interested in the world of herbal plants. Whether you are a budding herbalist, a healthcare professional, or simply someone curious about the natural world, this book aims to provide you with the knowledge and tools to identify, understand, and utilize herbal plants effectively.

What Are Herbal Plants?

- We begin our journey by exploring the essence of herbal plants. This chapter provides a foundational understanding of what constitutes an herbal plant, the various parts used, and their inherent medicinal properties.

Historical Significance of Herbal Plants

- Delve into the rich history of herbal medicine, tracing its roots from ancient civilizations to modern-day practices. This chapter highlights key historical figures, significant texts, and the evolution of herbal knowledge across different cultures.

Cultural Uses and Traditions

- Discover how various cultures around the world have used and continue to use herbal plants. From Indigenous traditions to Eastern and Western herbal practices, this chapter offers a global perspective on the cultural significance of herbal medicine.

Importance of Herbal Plants in Modern Medicine

- Examine the role of herbal plants in contemporary healthcare. This chapter discusses the integration of herbal remedies into modern medicine, supported by scientific research and clinical applications.

Botanical Descriptions

- Learn to identify herbal plants through detailed botanical descriptions. This chapter covers the morphology of leaves, stems, flowers, and roots, accompanied by high-quality photographs and illustrations for easy reference.

Principles of Plant Identification

- Equip yourself with the skills to accurately identify herbal plants. This chapter provides practical tips and techniques for distinguishing similar species, understanding seasonal variations, and recognizing key identification features.

Medicinal Uses and Benefits

- Explore the therapeutic properties of various herbal plants. This chapter includes comprehensive profiles of common herbs, detailing their medicinal uses, preparation methods, and benefits.

Safety and Toxicity Information

- Safety is paramount when using herbal plants. This chapter addresses potential side effects, contraindications, proper dosages, and guidelines for identifying and avoiding toxic look-alikes.

Cultivation and Harvesting

- Discover how to grow, harvest, and store herbal plants. This chapter provides practical advice on cultivating herbs in different environments, sustainable harvesting practices, and proper storage techniques to preserve their potency.

Recipes and Applications

- Put your knowledge into practice with a variety of recipes and applications. From herbal teas and tinctures to culinary uses and cosmetic preparations, this chapter offers step-by-step instructions to create your own herbal remedies.

Key Botanical Features for Identification

- Delve deeper into the botanical aspects of herbal plants. This chapter covers specific features such as leaf shapes, flower structures, stem characteristics, and sensory identifiers, enhancing your plant identification skills.

This book is not just a guide but an invitation to connect with nature, to understand the profound wisdom encoded in plants, and to embrace a holistic approach to health and well-being. As you embark on this journey, may you find inspiration, knowledge, and a deeper appreciation for the incredible world of herbal plants.

1

Botanical Descriptions

Botanical descriptions form the cornerstone of herbalism, offering a systematic approach to understanding and identifying medicinal plants. By meticulously documenting the morphology and characteristics of each plant, herbalists can confidently distinguish between species, assess their medicinal potential, and ensure accurate identification for safe and effective use.

Each part of the plant—the leaves, stems, flowers, and roots—holds valuable clues that reveal not only its identity but also its therapeutic properties. Detailed descriptions encompass not just physical attributes but also variations influenced by factors such as environment and growth stage. This knowledge allows herbalists to navigate the vast diversity of plant life with precision, unlocking the healing potential that nature offers.

In the pages that follow, we will explore the art and science of botanical descriptions. Through clear, detailed observations and illustrations, we aim to equip you with the essential skills to identify and appreciate herbal plants in their natural habitats. Whether you are a novice enthusiast or a seasoned practitioner, this chapter serves as a foundational guide to deepen your understanding of botanical diversity and its practical application in herbal medicine.

Morphology of Herbal Plants

In the intricate world of herbalism, the study of plant morphology is akin to deciphering nature's code—a detailed exploration that unveils the unique characteristics and potential of each botanical specimen. From the graceful sweep of leaves catching sunlight to the intricate network of roots delving deep into fertile soil, every aspect of a plant's morphology holds significance for herbalists seeking to harness its therapeutic benefits.

Leaves: Nature's Solar Collectors

- Leaves, with their myriad shapes, sizes, and textures, are the solar collectors of the plant world. They are not only vital for photosynthesis, the process by which plants convert sunlight into energy, but also integral to herbal medicine. The diverse forms of leaves—from delicate fern fronds to robust oak foliage—often hold clues to a plant's identity and medicinal properties.

- In herbalism, leaves are valued for their essential oils, tannins, and other bioactive compounds that contribute to their therapeutic effects. For instance, the broad, serrated leaves of ginkgo (Ginkgo biloba) are renowned for their cognitive-enhancing properties, while the heart-shaped leaves of hawthorn (Crataegus spp.) are prized for their cardiovascular benefits.

- The arrangement of leaves on a stem, known as phyllotaxy, varies widely among plants and provides important diagnostic information. Alternate leaves, such as those found on peppermint (Mentha × piperita), grow singly at different points along the stem. In contrast, opposite leaves, as seen in basil (Ocimum basilicum), emerge in pairs directly opposite each other on the stem. Whorled leaves, like those of Indian frankincense (Boswellia serrata), encircle the stem at regular intervals.

- Additionally, the margins or edges of leaves can be smooth, toothed, lobed, or deeply divided, further aiding in plant identification. The shape of the leaf blade—whether it is ovate (egg-shaped), lanceolate (lance-shaped), cordate (heart-shaped), or palmate (hand-shaped)—adds another layer of distinction. These botanical details, when carefully observed and recorded, enable herbalists to accurately identify and utilize plants in their practice.

Stems: Nature's Support Structures

- Stems serve as the architectural framework of plants, providing support for leaves, flowers, and fruits while transporting water, nutrients, and hormones throughout the organism. In herbal medicine, stems are less commonly used than leaves or roots but still hold medicinal potential, especially in certain traditions such as traditional Chinese medicine (TCM).

- The structure and growth habit of stems vary widely across plant species. Herbaceous plants, such as basil and parsley (Petroselinum crispum), have soft, green stems that are flexible and non-woody. These plants typically complete their life cycle within a single growing season. In contrast, woody plants like rosemary (Rosmarinus officinalis) and lavender (Lavandula spp.) develop hard, lignified stems that persist over multiple growing seasons, providing durability and structural integrity.

- Stem morphology includes characteristics such as texture (smooth, hairy, prickly), color (green, red, purple), and surface features (ridges, nodes, internodes). Nodes, where leaves, buds, or branches emerge from the stem, and internodes, the segments between nodes, are critical points of observation for herbalists. These features, along with stem growth patterns (erect, creeping, climbing), contribute to the overall identification and classification of plants.

Flowers: Nature's Beacons of Reproduction

- Flowers, with their vibrant colors, enticing scents, and intricate structures, are not merely ornamental but essential for a plant's reproductive success. Beyond their aesthetic appeal, flowers play a pivotal role in herbal medicine, offering a treasure trove of medicinal compounds that range from soothing chamomile (Matricaria chamomilla) to potent echinacea (Echinacea spp.).
- The morphology of flowers encompasses a multitude of features that aid in both identification and medicinal evaluation. The arrangement and number of flower parts—sepals, petals, stamens, and pistils—vary widely among plant families and species. For instance, members of the mint family (Lamiaceae) typically have bilaterally symmetrical flowers with four petals and four stamens, whereas members of the daisy family (Asteraceae) exhibit composite flower heads composed of numerous tiny florets.
- Flower color and scent are not merely aesthetic qualities but indicators of chemical constituents that contribute to medicinal properties. Brightly colored flowers, such as those of calendula (Calendula officinalis) and St. John's wort (Hypericum perforatum), often contain flavonoids and other antioxidants with anti-inflammatory and wound-healing properties. Fragrant flowers, like those of lavender and jasmine (Jasminum spp.), contain essential oils prized for their calming and mood-enhancing effects.
- Observing the arrangement of flowers on a plant—whether solitary, clustered into inflorescences, or arranged in panicles—provides additional diagnostic clues. The presence of nectar guides, patterns that direct pollinators toward the flower's reproductive structures, underscores the intricate co-evolutionary relationships between plants and their pollinators. Herbalists keenly observe these floral characteristics to identify plants accurately and determine their medicinal uses.

Roots: Nature's Anchors and Storehouses

- Roots are the hidden anchors that ground plants firmly in the soil, providing stability and absorbing water and nutrients essential for growth and survival. In herbal medicine, roots are prized for their concentrated stores of bioactive compounds, often harvested for their therapeutic effects on various bodily systems.

- Root morphology varies widely among plant species and reflects adaptations to different environments and growing conditions. Taproots, like those of dandelion (Taraxacum officinale), penetrate deep into the soil, anchoring the plant and accessing water and minerals from lower layers. Fibrous roots, characteristic of grasses and many herbaceous plants, form dense networks close to the soil surface, maximizing nutrient uptake in nutrient-poor environments.

- The external features of roots, such as color, texture, and branching patterns, provide important clues for identification. Medicinally valuable roots often exhibit distinct secondary growth features, including cambium layers and vascular tissues that transport nutrients throughout the plant. These structural adaptations contribute to the root's resilience and longevity, making them valuable sources of herbal medicine.

- Herbalists employ various methods for preparing and using roots in therapeutic formulations. Some roots, like ginger (Zingiber officinale) and turmeric (Curcuma longa), are dried and ground into powders for teas, tinctures, or capsules. Others, such as valerian (Valeriana officinalis) and licorice (Glycyrrhiza glabra), are decocted or infused to extract their beneficial compounds. Understanding root morphology and anatomy is essential for sustainable harvesting practices and ensuring the preservation of medicinal plant populations.

The morphology of herbal plants is a testament to the intricate adaptations and evolutionary strategies that plants have developed over millennia. By studying and understanding the leaves, stems, flowers, and roots of medicinal plants, herbalists gain profound insights into their identity, ecological roles, and therapeutic potentials. This chapter has provided a glimpse into the rich diversity of plant morphology and its significance in herbal medicine. As you continue your journey into the world of herbalism, may you find inspiration and appreciation for the botanical wonders that contribute to our health and well-being.

Growth Habits and Natural Habitats

The growth habits and natural habitats of herbal plants are a testament to their adaptability and ecological significance. Understanding where and how these plants thrive provides essential insights into their cultivation, harvesting, and conservation, ensuring sustainable practices that honor their medicinal potential and ecological roles.

Ecological Adaptations: Thriving in Diverse Environments

Herbal plants exhibit a remarkable diversity of growth habits, reflecting their adaptations to specific ecological niches and environmental conditions. These adaptations influence not only their physical appearance but also their biochemical composition and medicinal properties. From the sun-drenched slopes of Mediterranean cliffs to the shaded understory of temperate forests, each habitat shapes the growth habits and therapeutic potential of herbal plants.

1. Sun-loving Species: Plants adapted to sunny habitats, such as lavender (Lavandula spp.) and rosemary (Rosmarinus officinalis), thrive in well-drained soils with ample sunlight. Their compact growth forms and aromatic foliage are adaptations to arid conditions, where efficient water use and heat tolerance are essential for survival. These sun-loving herbs often produce essential oils rich in volatile compounds like terpenes and phenols, prized for their antimicrobial and antioxidant properties.

2. Shade-tolerant Species: In contrast, shade-tolerant herbs, such as ginseng (Panax spp.) and goldenseal (Hydrastis canadensis), flourish in the cool, dimly lit understory of deciduous forests. Their broad, thin leaves maximize light capture in low-light conditions, while their reliance on rich, moist soils underscores their preference for nutrient-rich habitats. These herbs often contain alkaloids and saponins that support immune function and enhance vitality, reflecting their adaptation to shaded environments.

3. Moisture-loving Species: Herbs that thrive in moist habitats, like marshmallow (Althaea officinalis) and watercress (Nasturtium officinale), are typically found along

riverbanks, wetlands, and boggy meadows. Their succulent leaves and water-absorbing roots are adaptations to fluctuating water levels, ensuring continuous nutrient uptake and growth. These moisture-loving plants often contain mucilage and polysaccharides that soothe and protect mucous membranes, making them valuable allies in respiratory and digestive health.

4. Arid-adapted Species: Plants adapted to arid environments, such as aloe vera (Aloe barbadensis) and prickly pear (Opuntia spp.), thrive in dry, sandy soils and endure prolonged periods of drought. Their fleshy leaves and water-storing tissues are adaptations that minimize water loss and maximize survival in water-limited habitats. These desert-dwelling herbs often produce gel-like substances and antioxidants that promote skin healing and hydration, reflecting their resilience in harsh climates.

Natural Habitats: Exploring Diversity and Conservation

The natural habitats of herbal plants encompass a tapestry of ecosystems, from mountainous slopes to coastal plains, each harboring unique species adapted to local climatic and soil conditions. These habitats provide not only a sanctuary for plant biodiversity but also essential resources for human health and well-being.

1. Forests and Woodlands: Forests and woodlands are rich reservoirs of herbal diversity, hosting species like elderberry (Sambucus nigra) and yarrow (Achillea millefolium). These habitats provide shade, moisture, and nutrient-rich soils that support the growth of medicinal plants with diverse ecological roles. Forest herbs often play crucial roles in ecosystem stability, contributing to soil fertility, water retention, and wildlife habitat.

2. Grasslands and Prairies: Grasslands and prairies are home to herbs like echinacea (Echinacea spp.) and milk thistle (Silybum marianum), adapted to open, sunlit environments with well-drained soils. These habitats support the growth of herbs with deep taproots that penetrate compacted soils and enhance nutrient cycling. Grassland herbs are often resilient to seasonal fluctuations in precipitation and temperature, reflecting their adaptation to semi-arid and continental climates.

3. **Wetlands and Riparian Zones:** Wetlands and riparian zones, such as marshes and riverbanks, nurture herbs like marshmallow and skullcap (Scutellaria spp.) that thrive in moist, nutrient-rich soils. These habitats play vital roles in water filtration, flood control, and habitat provision for aquatic and terrestrial species. Wetland herbs are often indicators of ecosystem health, reflecting water quality and nutrient cycling processes critical for ecological balance.

4. **Coastal and Mediterranean Environments:** Coastal and Mediterranean environments host herbs like thyme (Thymus vulgaris) and oregano (Origanum vulgare), adapted to sunny, well-drained soils with mild winters and dry summers. These habitats support herbs with aromatic foliage and essential oils that protect against salt spray and drought stress. Coastal herbs contribute to soil stabilization and erosion control, preserving coastal ecosystems vulnerable to climate change and human activities.

Conservation and Sustainable Practices

The conservation of herbal plants and their natural habitats is imperative to ensure their availability for future generations and to support biodiversity conservation efforts globally. Sustainable harvesting practices, cultivation initiatives, and habitat restoration projects are essential strategies to mitigate the impact of overharvesting, habitat loss, and climate change on medicinal plant populations.

Herbalists, botanists, and conservationists collaborate to promote ethical wildcrafting practices, which involve harvesting herbs in ways that minimize ecological impact and support plant regeneration. These practices include selecting mature plants, leaving sufficient individuals for natural propagation, and respecting seasonal growth cycles to preserve plant vitality and genetic diversity.

Cultivation of medicinal herbs in botanical gardens, community farms, and agroforestry systems provides alternative sources of herbal medicine while reducing pressure on wild populations. By cultivating endangered species like American ginseng and black cohosh (Actaea racemosa), herbalists contribute to conservation efforts and promote sustainable livelihoods for local communities.

Education and awareness initiatives play crucial roles in promoting the value of herbal plant conservation among consumers, healthcare professionals, and policymakers. Advocacy for policies that protect medicinal plant habitats, regulate trade in endangered species, and support sustainable herbal medicine practices is essential for the long-term conservation of plant biodiversity and ecosystem integrity.

The growth habits and natural habitats of herbal plants reveal their adaptive strategies, ecological roles, and potential contributions to human health and well-being. By understanding where and how these plants grow, herbalists gain insights into their cultivation, harvesting, and conservation, ensuring sustainable practices that honor their medicinal heritage and ecological significance. As stewards of nature's pharmacy, we are entrusted with preserving and nurturing herbal plant diversity for future generations, fostering a harmonious relationship between humans and the natural world.

Visual Aids: Photographs and Illustrations

Visual aids, such as photographs and illustrations, are invaluable tools in the world of herbalism, offering a window into the intricate beauty and medicinal potential of herbal plants. These visual representations serve multiple purposes, from aiding in plant identification and education to inspiring a deeper connection with nature's botanical wonders.

Capturing Nature's Beauty: The Art of Photography

Photographs of herbal plants capture more than just their physical appearance; they convey a sense of their natural habitat, seasonal variations, and growth stages. A well-composed photograph reveals the intricate details of leaves, stems, flowers, and roots, allowing herbalists to study botanical features with clarity and precision.

High-resolution images showcase the vibrant colors of flower petals, the intricate patterns of leaf veins, and the texture of bark and stems. These visual details are essential for distinguishing between similar species and verifying botanical characteristics critical for accurate identification. For example, close-up photographs of echinacea flowers highlight the distinctive cone-shaped center surrounded by vibrant pink petals, aiding in its recognition and differentiation from other daisy-like flowers.

Photographs also document the dynamic lifecycle of herbal plants, from seedling emergence to flowering and fruiting stages. Seasonal changes in foliage color and growth patterns provide insights into the plant's adaptation to environmental conditions and phenological cycles. By capturing these moments through photography, herbalists deepen their understanding of plant biology and ecological interactions, enriching their practice with nuanced observations.

Artistic Interpretations: Illustrating Botanical Beauty

Illustrations of herbal plants offer a blend of scientific accuracy and artistic interpretation, showcasing botanical details with a touch of creativity and aesthetic appeal. Botanical illustrators meticulously depict plant morphology, emphasizing key features essential for identification while infusing each illustration with a sense of botanical elegance.

Line drawings and watercolor paintings highlight the intricate structures of leaves, flowers, and roots, often accompanied by annotations that elucidate botanical terminology and functional characteristics. These illustrations serve as educational tools in botanical guides, herbal textbooks, and field manuals, providing visual references that transcend language barriers and enhance cross-cultural understanding of medicinal plants.

Illustrators bring to life the subtle nuances of plant diversity, from the delicate curl of a fern frond to the serrated edges of a mint leaf. By capturing these details in artful compositions, they evoke a sense of wonder and appreciation for the natural world, fostering a deeper connection between viewers and the plant kingdom.

Educational Value: Enhancing Learning and Appreciation

Visual aids play a pivotal role in herbal education, bridging theoretical knowledge with practical application in plant identification and medicinal uses. Educational posters, botanical atlases, and digital galleries compile a diverse array of photographs and illustrations, offering comprehensive visual catalogs of medicinal plants from around the globe.

These visual resources facilitate hands-on learning experiences for herbalists, students, and enthusiasts alike, enabling them to compare and contrast botanical features, study regional variations in plant morphology, and recognize cultural uses and medicinal traditions associated with specific herbs. Photographs of herbal preparations, such as dried leaves for tea or freshly harvested roots for tinctures, illustrate the diversity of herbal applications and processing techniques used in traditional and modern herbal medicine practices.

Beyond their educational utility, visual aids evoke an emotional response, sparking curiosity and admiration for the natural world's biodiversity. Photographs of sprawling meadows dotted with blooming chamomile or illustrations of ancient herbal gardens teeming with aromatic herbs evoke a sense of reverence for traditional knowledge and ecological stewardship. These visual narratives inspire a commitment to conservation efforts and sustainable practices that safeguard herbal plant diversity for future generations.

Visual aids—whether through photographs capturing nature's beauty or illustrations interpreting botanical elegance—are essential companions in the journey of herbalism. They illuminate the intricate details and ecological adaptations of herbal plants, enriching our understanding of their medicinal potential and cultural significance. As we embrace the art and science of herbalism, may these visual representations continue to inspire awe, deepen our connection with nature, and foster a legacy of stewardship that preserves herbal plant diversity for generations to come.

2

Principles of Plant Identification

The principles of plant identification form the bedrock of herbalism, providing a systematic framework for discerning and understanding the diverse array of medicinal plants that grace our planet. Rooted in botany and enriched by centuries of traditional knowledge, these principles empower herbalists to navigate the intricacies of plant taxonomy, morphology, and ecological adaptations with precision and confidence.

Plant identification begins with keen observation—scrutinizing the unique features of leaves, stems, flowers, and roots that distinguish one species from another. By documenting these botanical characteristics in detail, herbalists unravel the botanical mysteries that define each plant's identity and medicinal potential.

Beyond morphology, plant identification embraces ecological contexts—studying habitats, growth habits, and environmental preferences that shape a plant's life cycle and distribution. This holistic approach connects herbalists to the natural rhythms and ecological niches that sustain medicinal plant populations, guiding ethical harvesting practices and conservation efforts.

In the chapters that follow, we delve into the principles that underpin plant identification, from the nuanced complexities of botanical taxonomy to practical field techniques for accurate species recognition. By mastering these principles, herbalists embark on a journey of discovery, forging deeper connections with the plant kingdom and harnessing nature's healing gifts with reverence and respect.

Key Features for Identification

In the pursuit of plant identification, attention to key botanical features is paramount. These features serve as the guiding compass, steering herbalists through the labyrinth of plant diversity and facilitating accurate species recognition. By honing their observational skills and understanding the significance of these features, herbalists unlock the door to a world rich in medicinal potential and ecological wonder.

Leaves

Leaves are often the first chapter in the story of plant identification, offering a wealth of information through their size, shape, arrangement, and surface characteristics. The morphology of leaves varies widely among plant species, from the needle-like leaves of conifers to the broad, lobed leaves of maple trees.

1. Leaf Shape and Margins: The shape of a leaf—whether it is ovate, lanceolate, cordate, or palmate—provides initial clues to a plant's identity. Similarly, the margins of leaves—whether they are smooth, serrated, lobed, or toothed—offer further diagnostic information. For instance, the finely toothed margins of mint leaves distinguish them from the deeply lobed leaves of oak trees.

2. Leaf Arrangement: The arrangement of leaves along the stem—whether they are alternate, opposite, or whorled—adds another layer of identification. Alternate leaves, such as those of rosemary and basil, grow singly at different points along the stem. Opposite leaves, as seen in elderberry and ash trees, emerge in pairs directly opposite each other. Whorled leaves encircle the stem at regular intervals, as observed in plants like pineapples and some cacti.

3. Leaf Surface Characteristics: The surface texture of leaves—whether they are smooth, hairy, glossy, or textured—provides additional clues for identification. For example, the velvety texture of lamb's ear leaves contrasts with the waxy, glossy surface of holly leaves. Observing these surface characteristics under varying light conditions can reveal subtle details that aid in distinguishing between closely related species.

Stems and Bark:

Stems and bark serve as structural foundations that support plant growth and transport vital nutrients throughout the organism. The morphology of stems—whether they are herbaceous or woody, erect or climbing—reflects adaptations to different environmental conditions and growth habits.

1. Stem Texture and Color: The texture of stems—whether they are smooth, rough, hairy, or prickly—provides tactile clues for identification. Similarly, stem color—ranging from green to brown, red, or purple—varies among plant species and can be influenced by factors such as age, sunlight exposure, and seasonal changes.

2. Bark Characteristics: In woody plants, the bark serves as a protective outer layer that insulates against environmental stresses and physical damage. Bark characteristics—such as texture (smooth, rough, fissured), color (light, dark, mottled), and pattern—offer diagnostic features for species identification. For example, the distinctive peeling bark of

paperbark maple (Acer griseum) contrasts with the deeply furrowed bark of white oak (Quercus alba).

Flowers and Inflorescences

Flowers and inflorescences are nature's masterpieces, showcasing a dazzling array of colors, shapes, and fragrances that attract pollinators and ensure reproductive success. The morphology of flowers—whether they are solitary, clustered into inflorescences, or arranged in dense spikes—provides essential clues for plant identification and medicinal evaluation.

1. Flower Structure: The structure of flowers—comprising sepals, petals, stamens, and pistils—varies widely among plant families and species. Observing the number, arrangement, and fusion of these floral parts aids in distinguishing between different types of flowers. For instance, the tubular flowers of foxglove (Digitalis purpurea) are characteristic of plants in the figwort family (Scrophulariaceae), whereas the composite flower heads of sunflowers (Helianthus annuus) consist of numerous tiny florets.

2. Inflorescence Types: The arrangement of flowers on a plant—whether they are borne singly, in clusters, or in dense spikes—provides additional diagnostic information. Inflorescence types include racemes, panicles, umbels, and spikes, each with unique characteristics that aid in species recognition. For example, the compact umbels of dill (Anethum graveolens) distinguish it from the elongated spikes of lavender (Lavandula spp.).

Roots and Rhizomes

Roots and rhizomes are the hidden treasures of herbal plants, harboring concentrated stores of bioactive compounds essential for medicinal purposes. The morphology of roots—whether they are fibrous, taprooted, or tuberous—reflects adaptations to different soil types and growth conditions. These underground structures provide resilience and longevity, supporting the plant's survival and ecological fitness.

1. Root Structure: The structure of roots—comprising primary roots, lateral roots, and root hairs—facilitates nutrient uptake and water absorption from the soil. Observing root characteristics such as color, texture, and branching patterns provides crucial information for species identification. For example, the distinctive yellow color and spicy aroma of

turmeric (Curcuma longa) roots contrast with the fibrous, white roots of horseradish (Armoracia rusticana).

2. Rhizome Characteristics: Rhizomes are horizontal underground stems that store nutrients and produce new shoots and roots. The morphology of rhizomes—whether they are thickened or slender, segmented or continuous—varies among plant species and influences their growth habits and medicinal properties. For example, the knobby rhizomes of ginger (Zingiber officinale) are prized for their spicy flavor and digestive benefits, while the creeping rhizomes of goldenseal (Hydrastis canadensis) contain berberine alkaloids with antimicrobial properties.

Tips for Distinguishing Similar Species

In the intricate world of plant identification, distinguishing between similar species requires careful observation, attention to detail, and a nuanced understanding of botanical characteristics. Similar species often share overlapping features that challenge herbalists to discern subtle differences that may impact medicinal efficacy and safety.

1. Comparative Analysis: Compare multiple specimens of the same species and closely related species side by side. Note differences in leaf shape, size, arrangement, and texture, as well as variations in stem characteristics and flower morphology. A comparative approach enhances visual memory and facilitates recognition of diagnostic features that distinguish one species from another.

2. Seasonal Variations: Observe plants throughout their lifecycle and note seasonal changes in foliage, flower color, and fruit development. Many plants exhibit distinct phenological stages—such as leaf emergence in spring, flowering in summer, and fruiting in autumn—that provide additional clues for identification. Seasonal variations in growth habit and habitat preference further refine species differentiation and enhance accuracy in plant recognition.

3. Ecological Context: Consider the ecological context in which plants are found, including habitat preferences, soil types, and associated plant communities. Plants adapted to specific environments—such as wetlands, woodlands, or

coastal dunes—often exhibit unique adaptations and growth habits that distinguish them from similar species in other habitats. Understanding these ecological nuances informs species identification and enhances appreciation for the interconnectedness of plants within their natural communities.

4. **Use of Botanical Keys:** Consult botanical keys, field guides, and taxonomic resources that provide detailed descriptions and illustrations of plant characteristics. Botanical keys employ dichotomous or descriptive criteria to guide users through a series of paired choices based on observable features, leading to the identification of unknown plant specimens. These resources serve as invaluable tools for validating identification hypotheses and refining species differentiation in diverse plant communities.

5. **Seek Expert Guidance:** Seek guidance from experienced herbalists, botanists, and local plant experts who possess specialized knowledge of regional flora and medicinal plants. Engage in field-based learning experiences, workshops, and botanical expeditions that foster hands-on skills in plant identification and deepen understanding of plant diversity. Collaboration with knowledgeable mentors enriches learning opportunities and cultivates a passion for lifelong exploration of herbal plants and their ecological significance.

The principles of plant identification and tips for distinguishing similar species form the cornerstone of herbalism, empowering practitioners to navigate the complexities of plant taxonomy and morphology with precision and confidence. By mastering these principles and refining observational skills, herbalists deepen their connection with medicinal plants and uphold ethical practices that honor biodiversity conservation and sustainable herbal medicine. As stewards of nature's pharmacy, we embrace the art and science of plant identification with reverence, recognizing the profound role of botanical diversity in promoting health, well-being, and ecological harmony.

Seasonal Variations and Growth Stages

The lifecycle of herbal plants unfolds in rhythmic harmony with the changing seasons, each phase marked by distinct physiological transitions and adaptive strategies that optimize growth, reproduction, and survival.

Seasonal variations and growth stages offer a window into the dynamic nature of plant biology, illuminating the interplay between environmental cues, biological rhythms, and medicinal potency.

Embracing Nature's Rhythms: Seasonal Transitions

Herbal plants exhibit profound seasonal variations in response to environmental cues such as temperature, daylight duration, and precipitation patterns. These seasonal transitions influence phenological events—such as bud burst, flowering, fruiting, and dormancy—that synchronize plant growth with optimal conditions for pollination, seed dispersal, and nutrient acquisition.

1. **Spring Awakening:** As winter recedes and daylight lengthens, herbal plants emerge from dormancy with renewed vigor. Spring heralds the awakening of dormant buds and the emergence of tender shoots adorned with fresh foliage. Early-flowering species, such as dandelion (Taraxacum officinale) and nettle (Urtica dioica), seize the opportunity to bloom, attracting pollinators and replenishing energy reserves stored in roots and rhizomes during winter dormancy.
2. **Summer Splendor:** Summer represents a season of abundance and growth for herbal plants, characterized by lush foliage, vibrant flowers, and prolific seed production. Long daylight hours and warm temperatures accelerate photosynthesis and metabolic processes, fueling rapid vegetative growth and reproductive success. Herbs like chamomile (Matricaria chamomilla) and lemon balm (Melissa officinalis) thrive in the summer sun, harnessing solar energy to synthesize essential oils and bioactive compounds that enhance medicinal potency.
3. **Autumn Harvest:** As daylight wanes and temperatures cool, herbal plants undergo physiological changes that prepare them for winter dormancy and seed dispersal. Autumn foliage transitions from green to hues of red, orange, and yellow, signaling the accumulation of nutrients in roots, rhizomes, and seeds. Medicinal plants such as echinacea (Echinacea purpurea) and garlic (Allium sativum) reach peak potency as they store bioactive compounds essential for immune support and winter resilience.
4. **Winter Rest:** Winter imposes a period of dormancy and metabolic slowdown for many herbal plants, conserving

energy and protecting against freezing temperatures. Deciduous species shed their leaves, while perennial herbs withdraw vital nutrients into underground storage organs like roots, rhizomes, and bulbs. Dormant buds await the signal of spring's return, poised to initiate new growth and resume the seasonal cycle of renewal.

Growth Stages

The growth stages of herbal plants unfold through a sequence of developmental milestones that reflect physiological maturity, reproductive readiness, and adaptation to environmental challenges. From seed germination to senescence, each growth stage offers insights into plant vigor, resilience, and medicinal potential shaped by genetic predisposition and environmental interactions.

1. Germination and Seedling Establishment: The journey of an herbal plant begins with seed germination—a transformative process triggered by favorable soil moisture, temperature, and light conditions. Germinating seeds develop into seedlings equipped with cotyledons (seed leaves) that nourish early growth and establish root systems essential for nutrient uptake and water absorption. Seedling establishment marks the foundation of plant growth, setting the stage for vegetative development and reproductive success.

2. Vegetative Growth: During the vegetative growth stage, herbal plants allocate energy towards leaf expansion, stem elongation, and root proliferation. Photosynthesis fuels the synthesis of carbohydrates, proteins, and secondary metabolites that support cellular functions and structural integrity. Leafy herbs like parsley (Petroselinum crispum) and comfrey (Symphytum officinale) exhibit vigorous vegetative growth, producing abundant foliage rich in chlorophyll and essential nutrients essential for culinary and medicinal applications.

3. Reproductive Phase: The reproductive phase marks a transformative milestone in the lifecycle of herbal plants, culminating in the production of flowers, fruits, and seeds essential for genetic diversity and species propagation. Floral buds develop into intricate blooms adorned with petals, stamens, and pistils that facilitate pollination and fertilization. Pollinators—such as bees, butterflies, and hummingbirds—play pivotal roles in transferring pollen

between flowers, ensuring successful seed set and fruit development. Herbs like milk thistle (Silybum marianum) and evening primrose (Oenothera biennis) showcase striking flowers that attract pollinators and yield nutrient-rich seeds prized for their medicinal properties.

4. Senescence and Dormancy: As herbal plants complete their reproductive cycle, senescence initiates physiological changes that prepare for dormancy and winter survival. Mature leaves yellow and senesce, diverting nutrients from foliage to roots and storage organs like rhizomes and tubers. Dormant buds encased in protective scales await the onset of favorable conditions, poised to initiate new growth and rejuvenate the plant in the coming seasons. Perennial herbs such as valerian (Valeriana officinalis) and ginseng (Panax spp.) exhibit dormancy strategies that conserve energy and ensure longevity, adapting to seasonal fluctuations in temperature and moisture availability.

Seasonal variations and growth stages embody the cyclical rhythms and transformative resilience of herbal plants, unveiling the interconnectedness of botanical life with environmental dynamics. By embracing nature's seasonal cues and observing growth stages with reverence, herbalists deepen their understanding of plant biology and medicinal potency, fostering a holistic approach to herbal medicine that honors ecological stewardship and sustainable practices. As we navigate the seasonal ebb and flow of herbal plants, may we cultivate a profound appreciation for their resilience, adaptability, and timeless contributions to human health and well-being.

3

Medicinal Uses and Benefits

Medicinal uses and benefits lie at the heart of herbalism, weaving together centuries of traditional wisdom, scientific inquiry, and holistic approaches to health and wellness. Herbal plants have long been revered for their therapeutic properties, offering a diverse array of bioactive compounds that support the body's natural healing processes and promote overall well-being.

From ancient civilizations to modern herbal medicine practices, plants have served as invaluable sources of medicine, providing remedies for ailments ranging from minor discomforts to chronic conditions. The medicinal potential of herbal plants is vast, encompassing a spectrum of applications that address physiological, emotional, and spiritual dimensions of health.

In exploring the medicinal uses and benefits of herbal plants, we embark on a journey of discovery—one that bridges ancient traditions with contemporary research, fostering a deeper appreciation for nature's pharmacy and its profound impact on human health. Through systematic exploration and evidence-based practice, herbalists harness the therapeutic power of plants to nurture vitality, resilience, and balance in individuals and communities alike.

In the chapters that follow, we delve into the multifaceted realm of medicinal plants, exploring their diverse therapeutic actions, traditional uses, and scientific insights that underpin their efficacy. By embracing the rich tapestry of herbal medicine, we honor a legacy of healing that transcends cultural boundaries and celebrates the inherent wisdom of nature's botanical treasures.

Common and Scientific Names

1. **Common Names:** Common names of medicinal plants reflect cultural heritage, regional traditions, and practical applications ingrained in local communities over generations. These vernacular names often evoke the plant's appearance, aroma, taste, or historical uses, fostering a deep connection between people and the natural world. For instance, the common name "St. John's wort" (Hypericum perforatum) honors its traditional harvesting on St. John's Day (June 24) and underscores its association with mental health and well-being.

2. **Scientific Names:** Scientific names, or binomial nomenclature, provide a universal language for botanical classification based on genus and species. Established by Carl Linnaeus

in the 18th century, this standardized system ensures clarity and accuracy in identifying and categorizing plant species worldwide. The genus name (e.g., Hypericum) denotes a group of closely related species, while the species epithet (e.g., perforatum) distinguishes a specific plant within the genus. Scientific names transcend linguistic and cultural barriers, enabling precise communication among herbalists, botanists, and researchers engaged in plant taxonomy and medicinal research.

Traditional Uses

Ethnobotanical Insights

- Traditional uses of medicinal plants embody millennia of ethnobotanical knowledge passed down through oral traditions, rituals, and healing practices of indigenous cultures worldwide. These cultural legacies illuminate the diverse therapeutic applications of plants, ranging from culinary herbs used to enhance digestion to sacred botanicals revered for spiritual healing and ceremonial rites. Ethnobotanical studies document the profound role of plants in addressing community health needs, sustaining cultural identity, and preserving ecological wisdom integral to sustainable livelihoods.

Global Traditions

- Across continents and climates, traditional herbalism embraces a tapestry of botanical diversity, each plant celebrated for its unique healing virtues rooted in local ecosystems and ancestral wisdom. In Ayurveda, the ancient healing tradition of India, herbs such as turmeric (Curcuma longa) and holy basil (Ocimum sanctum) are revered for their holistic benefits in balancing doshas (bioenergetic forces) and promoting longevity. Similarly, Traditional Chinese Medicine (TCM) integrates herbs like ginseng (Panax ginseng) and astragalus (Astragalus membranaceus) to harmonize qi (vital energy) and restore harmony between body, mind, and spirit.

European Herbalism

- European herbalism traces its lineage to classical antiquity, where herbs like chamomile (Matricaria chamomilla) and valerian (Valeriana officinalis) were esteemed for their calming properties and digestive support. Medieval monastic gardens cultivated a wealth of medicinal herbs, including rosemary (Rosmarinus officinalis) and sage (Salvia officinalis), cherished for their culinary uses and therapeutic benefits in treating ailments ranging from headaches to respiratory infections. The Renaissance era witnessed a resurgence of botanical exploration and herbal knowledge, as herbalists and botanists cataloged newfound species and expanded the pharmacopeia of medicinal plants.

Modern Applications

Scientific Validation

- Modern applications of medicinal plants integrate traditional wisdom with rigorous scientific inquiry, exploring phytochemical profiles, pharmacological mechanisms, and clinical efficacy to validate therapeutic claims and inform evidence-based practice. Phytochemistry elucidates the chemical composition of plants, identifying bioactive compounds—such as alkaloids, flavonoids, and terpenes—that contribute to their medicinal properties. Pharmacological studies assess the physiological effects of plant extracts and isolated compounds, elucidating mechanisms of action and potential therapeutic targets in treating diverse health conditions.

Herbal Medicine Practices

- Herbal medicine practices encompass diverse modalities, from herbal teas and tinctures to botanical supplements and topical preparations, tailored to individual health needs and therapeutic goals. Herbalists collaborate with healthcare providers to integrate botanical therapies into holistic treatment plans, promoting wellness, disease prevention, and patient-centered care. Integrative medicine approaches combine conventional treatments with evidence-based herbal interventions, fostering synergy between medical disciplines and enhancing patient outcomes in managing chronic conditions such as cardiovascular disease, diabetes, and autoimmune disorders.

Nutritional and Culinary Uses

- Beyond medicinal applications, herbal plants enrich culinary traditions and dietary practices, enhancing flavor profiles, and nutritional value in culinary preparations. Culinary herbs like basil (Ocimum basilicum) and cilantro (Coriandrum sativum) infuse dishes with aromatic nuances and essential nutrients that support digestive health and culinary creativity. Herbal teas and infusions— such as peppermint (Mentha × piperita) and chamomile— soothe the senses and promote relaxation, offering therapeutic benefits beyond their culinary appeal.

The exploration of common and scientific names, traditional uses, and modern applications of medicinal plants illuminates a continuum of human interaction with botanical diversity, from ancient healing traditions to contemporary integrative medicine practices. By honoring cultural heritage, embracing scientific inquiry, and fostering holistic approaches to health and wellness, we cultivate a deeper appreciation for the therapeutic potential of plants and their enduring legacy in promoting vitality, resilience, and harmony within individuals and communities worldwide. As we navigate the evolving landscape of herbal medicine, may we continue to uphold principles of sustainability, ethical stewardship, and cultural diversity that safeguard the future of plant-based healing for generations to come.

Preparation Methods

Herbal Teas

Herbal teas, also known as infusions or tisanes, embody the art and science of extracting medicinal properties from plants through steeping in hot water. This time-honored method dates back centuries, offering a soothing and palatable way to imbibe the therapeutic benefits of herbs. Whether enjoyed hot or cold, herbal teas provide a gentle and effective means to support digestion, promote relaxation, and enhance overall well-being.

1. Brewing Techniques: Brewing herbal teas involves steeping dried or fresh herbs in hot water for a specified duration to extract bioactive compounds and aromatic oils. The ideal water temperature and steeping time vary depending on the herb's delicate constituents and desired therapeutic effects. For example, delicate herbs like chamomile (Matricaria chamomilla) benefit from lower temperatures and shorter steeping times to preserve

volatile oils and maximize flavor.

2. Health Benefits: Herbal teas offer a spectrum of health benefits tailored to individual needs and preferences. Peppermint tea (Mentha × piperita), prized for its refreshing taste and digestive properties, alleviates nausea, bloating, and indigestion. Ginger tea (Zingiber officinale) warms the body, stimulates circulation, and eases symptoms of colds and flu. Lemon balm tea (Melissa officinalis) calms the mind, reduces stress, and promotes restful sleep. Regular consumption of herbal teas supports hydration, encourages detoxification, and nurtures holistic well-being through daily rituals of self-care.

Tinctures

Tinctures represent potent herbal extracts crafted through the maceration of plant material in alcohol or glycerin, harnessing the concentrated essence of medicinal plants. This extraction method enhances bioavailability and shelf stability, facilitating precise dosage and therapeutic efficacy in addressing a myriad of health concerns. Tinctures offer a versatile and convenient approach to herbal supplementation, supporting immune function, enhancing vitality, and promoting resilience during times of physical and emotional stress.

1. Extraction Process: The tincture-making process begins with selecting high-quality herbs rich in active constituents such as alkaloids, flavonoids, and essential oils. Plant material is finely chopped or ground to optimize surface area for extraction, then macerated in alcohol (e.g., ethanol or vodka) or glycerin to facilitate the release and dissolution of bioactive compounds. The maceration period varies from several days to weeks, allowing time for the solvent to extract and concentrate herbal constituents.

2. Dosage and Administration: Tinctures offer flexible dosage options tailored to individual health needs and therapeutic goals. Herbalists recommend precise dosages based on herb potency, desired effects, and individual sensitivity. Tinctures may be taken orally by diluting drops in water or juice, facilitating rapid absorption and systemic distribution of medicinal compounds. Sublingual administration—placing drops under the tongue—enhances bioavailability and accelerates onset of therapeutic action, ideal for acute conditions requiring immediate relief.

3. **Therapeutic Applications:** Tinctures support diverse therapeutic applications, from immune modulation and stress management to digestive support and hormonal balance. Echinacea tincture (Echinacea purpurea) strengthens immune defenses, offering protection against respiratory infections and seasonal allergies. St. John's wort tincture (Hypericum perforatum) uplifts mood, alleviates symptoms of depression, and supports emotional well-being. Milk thistle tincture (Silybum marianum) promotes liver detoxification, enhancing metabolic function and protecting against oxidative stress. Regular use of tinctures fosters resilience, vitality, and holistic equilibrium, promoting sustainable health practices rooted in nature's botanical wisdom.

Poultices

Poultices embody the therapeutic art of applying fresh or dried herbs directly to the skin as compresses or pastes, harnessing nature's healing properties to alleviate pain, reduce inflammation, and promote tissue regeneration. This ancient healing modality offers localized relief and systemic benefits, enhancing circulation, accelerating wound healing, and restoring balance to musculoskeletal and dermal systems.

1. **Preparation Techniques:** Crafting a poultice begins with selecting herbs renowned for their anti-inflammatory, analgesic, and antimicrobial properties. Fresh or dried plant material—such as comfrey (Symphytum officinale), calendula (Calendula officinalis), or turmeric (Curcuma longa)—is finely chopped or ground to form a cohesive paste. The herbal paste is applied directly to affected areas of the body, covered with a clean cloth or bandage to retain moisture and facilitate herbal absorption.

2. **Therapeutic Benefits:** Poultices offer targeted relief for acute injuries, chronic pain, and inflammatory conditions affecting muscles, joints, and skin. Arnica poultice (Arnica montana) reduces bruising and swelling, accelerating recovery from sports injuries and trauma. Plantain poultice (Plantago major) soothes insect bites, rashes, and minor burns, providing immediate relief and promoting tissue repair. Mustard seed poultice stimulates circulation, alleviating congestion, and supporting respiratory function during colds and respiratory infections. Regular application of poultices enhances local circulation, reduces discomfort, and supports

natural healing processes, fostering optimal recovery and functional restoration.

Preparation methods such as herbal teas, tinctures, and poultices exemplify the artistry and efficacy of herbal medicine in promoting health, resilience, and holistic well-being. Through meticulous extraction techniques and application practices, herbalists harness nature's botanical treasures to address diverse health concerns, from everyday ailments to chronic conditions requiring comprehensive therapeutic support.

By integrating traditional wisdom with modern scientific inquiry, herbal medicine continues to evolve as a vital component of integrative healthcare, empowering individuals to cultivate vitality, balance, and harmony through sustainable practices rooted in nature's timeless wisdom. As we explore the multifaceted benefits of herbal preparations, may we honor the interconnectedness of human health with ecological stewardship, fostering a future where botanical diversity thrives and healing flourishes for generations to come.

4

Safety and Toxicity Information

Safety and toxicity considerations are paramount in the practice of herbal medicine, ensuring the responsible use of botanical remedies to promote health and minimize potential risks. Herbalists and healthcare practitioners navigate a complex landscape of plant constituents, dosage guidelines, and individual susceptibility factors to safeguard patient well-being and optimize therapeutic outcomes. Understanding the principles of safety and toxicity empowers practitioners to make informed decisions, cultivate trust with clients, and uphold ethical standards in herbal practice.

Herbal medicine embraces a rich tapestry of botanical diversity, each plant imbued with unique therapeutic properties and chemical constituents that contribute to its medicinal efficacy. However, alongside the benefits, herbs possess inherent complexities, including the potential for adverse reactions, interactions with medications, and variability in potency due to cultivation, processing, and individual response.

By integrating safety protocols, evidence-based assessments, and ongoing education, herbalists mitigate risks and foster a holistic approach to patient care rooted in integrity, compassion, and sustainable health practices.

In the chapters that follow, we explore the intricacies of safety and toxicity in herbal medicine, examining pharmacological principles, regulatory standards, and clinical considerations that inform responsible prescribing, patient counseling, and therapeutic monitoring. By promoting transparency, accountability, and collaboration across healthcare disciplines, we uphold a commitment to patient safety, respect diverse cultural traditions, and advance the integration of herbal medicine within contemporary healthcare frameworks. As stewards of botanical wisdom, we embrace the imperative to balance innovation with precaution, ensuring that the therapeutic potential of herbs aligns harmoniously with principles of safety, efficacy, and holistic wellness.

Potential Side Effects and Contraindications

Understanding Side Effects

Potential side effects of herbal medicines encompass a spectrum of physiological responses that may occur when using botanical remedies. These effects can vary widely depending on the herb's potency, dosage, individual sensitivity, and duration of use. Common side effects may include gastrointestinal disturbances, allergic reactions, skin irritations, and changes in physiological functions such as blood pressure or heart rate. Herbalists employ comprehensive intake assessments, including medical history, allergies, and concurrent medications, to mitigate risks and tailor treatment plans to individual health needs.

1. **Adverse Reactions:** Certain herbs may elicit adverse reactions in susceptible individuals, manifesting as nausea, headaches, dizziness, or mild gastrointestinal discomfort. For example, excessive consumption of licorice root (Glycyrrhiza glabra) may elevate blood pressure and cause potassium depletion, posing risks for individuals with hypertension or cardiac conditions. Allergic responses to herbs like chamomile (Matricaria chamomilla) or echinacea (Echinacea purpurea) may manifest as skin rashes, itching, or respiratory symptoms in sensitive individuals. Vigilance in monitoring symptoms and adjusting herbal formulations ensures safe and effective therapeutic outcomes while minimizing potential adverse effects.

2. **Herb-Drug Interactions:** Herb-drug interactions present a critical consideration in herbal medicine practice, involving the modulation of drug metabolism, absorption, or excretion pathways that impact therapeutic efficacy and safety. St. John's wort (Hypericum perforatum), renowned for its antidepressant properties, induces cytochrome P450 enzymes responsible for metabolizing medications such as selective serotonin reuptake inhibitors (SSRIs), oral contraceptives, and anticoagulants. Concurrent use of herbs with anticoagulant properties, such as ginkgo (Ginkgo biloba) or garlic (Allium sativum), may potentiate bleeding risks and necessitate cautious monitoring in patients on antithrombotic therapy. Herbalists collaborate with healthcare providers to navigate complex interactions, optimize treatment regimens, and promote patient-centered care that integrates conventional and botanical therapies effectively.

Contraindications: Safety Precautions and Health Considerations

Contraindications in herbal medicine denote conditions or circumstances where specific herbs pose potential risks or are unsuitable for use due to physiological, pharmacological, or therapeutic implications. These contraindications inform clinical decision-making and treatment planning, ensuring patient safety and mitigating adverse outcomes.

Herbalists conduct thorough assessments and educate clients on contraindications relevant to their health status, empowering informed choices and promoting responsible self-care practices.

1. Pregnancy and Lactation: Pregnancy and lactation impose unique considerations in herbal medicine practice, as certain herbs may exert uterotonic effects, alter hormone levels, or cross the placental barrier, potentially impacting fetal development or breastfeeding infants. Herbs like black cohosh (Actaea racemosa) and pennyroyal (Mentha pulegium) are contraindicated during pregnancy due to their potential to induce uterine contractions and adverse fetal outcomes. Safe alternatives such as ginger (Zingiber officinale) for nausea or raspberry leaf (Rubus idaeus) for uterine toning require careful evaluation and guidance from qualified healthcare providers to support maternal health and well-being.

2. Pre-existing Health Conditions: Pre-existing health conditions—such as liver disease, kidney dysfunction, cardiovascular disorders, or autoimmune conditions—may influence herb selection, dosing strategies, and treatment outcomes in herbal medicine practice. Herbs with hepatotoxic potential, such as kava (Piper methysticum) or comfrey (Symphytum officinale), warrant caution and monitoring in individuals with compromised liver function to prevent exacerbation of symptoms or adverse hepatic effects. Similarly, herbs that affect renal function, such as juniper berry (Juniperus communis) or parsley (Petroselinum crispum), require individualized dosing considerations and vigilant assessment of renal function markers to ensure safe and effective therapeutic outcomes.

Proper Dosages and Usage Guidelines

Individualized Dosage Considerations

Proper dosages and usage guidelines in herbal medicine emphasize personalized care and evidence-based practice to optimize therapeutic efficacy while minimizing potential risks and adverse effects. Herbalists employ dosage titration, therapeutic monitoring, and client education to support safe and effective use of botanical remedies tailored to individual health needs, preferences, and treatment goals.

1. **Dosage Titration:** Dosage titration involves gradual adjustment of herbal formulations to achieve therapeutic effects while mitigating risks of adverse reactions or sensitivities. Initial dosages consider factors such as age, weight, metabolic rate, and overall health status to establish a baseline for therapeutic response and tolerance. Herbalists monitor client responses closely, adjusting dosages based on symptom alleviation, biochemical markers, and subjective feedback to optimize treatment outcomes and promote long-term health benefits.

2. **Duration of Use:** Duration of herbal use varies depending on the herb's therapeutic indication, treatment goals, and individual response. Short-term use of herbs like echinacea (Echinacea purpurea) for immune support during acute infections or seasonal allergies ensures efficacy without compromising immune resilience or inducing tolerance. Chronic conditions requiring long-term herbal support—such as cardiovascular health, joint inflammation, or metabolic disorders—incorporate periodic breaks or rotational therapies to prevent adaptation, enhance therapeutic response, and maintain herbal efficacy over time.

3. **Quality and Standardization:** Herbal quality and standardization ensure consistency, potency, and safety in botanical preparations, supporting reliable therapeutic outcomes and consumer confidence. Certified organic cultivation practices, sustainable harvesting methods, and stringent quality control measures safeguard herbal integrity, minimizing contaminants, adulterants, and variability in bioactive constituents. Standardized herbal extracts—validated through phytochemical analysis and pharmacological profiling—provide consistent dosages of active compounds, facilitating precise therapeutic dosing and clinical efficacy in herbal medicine practice.

Potential side effects, contraindications, proper dosages, and usage guidelines underscore the principles of safety, efficacy, and patient-centered care in herbal medicine practice. By integrating evidence-based assessments, individualized treatment plans, and collaborative healthcare strategies, herbalists promote optimal therapeutic outcomes, enhance patient safety, and foster a culture of responsible self-care rooted in botanical wisdom. As stewards of holistic health, we uphold ethical standards, advocate for informed decision-making, and advance the integration of herbal medicine within comprehensive healthcare frameworks that prioritize integrity, compassion, and sustainable wellness for all individuals and communities. Through ongoing education, research advancements, and shared dialogue, we celebrate the transformative potential of herbs as allies in promoting vitality, resilience, and holistic well-being across the lifespan.

Identifying Toxic Look-Alikes

Importance of Plant Identification

Identifying toxic look-alikes is critical in herbal medicine to prevent inadvertent ingestion of harmful plants that resemble beneficial botanicals in appearance, habitat, or growth habits. Accurate plant identification relies on botanical knowledge, taxonomic expertise, and practical field experience to distinguish between species with similar morphological characteristics but distinct chemical compositions or toxicological profiles. Herbalists employ rigorous assessment protocols, botanical keys, and consultation with botanical experts to ensure safety, mitigate risks, and uphold ethical standards in herbal practice.

1. Morphological Features: Morphological features—including leaf shape, stem structure, flower morphology, and fruit characteristics—serve as primary indicators for differentiating between herbal plants and their toxic counterparts. For example, the distinct white berries and glossy, alternate leaves of deadly nightshade (Atropa belladonna) contrast with the edible black berries and serrated, compound leaves of elderberry (Sambucus nigra). Detailed botanical descriptions, comparative analysis, and hands-on training enhance proficiency in plant recognition and reduce the likelihood of misidentification in natural habitats or cultivated landscapes.

2. Habitat and Ecological Niche: Habitat and ecological niche provide contextual clues for identifying plant species and discerning potential toxic look-alikes within specific geographic regions or ecological communities. Poison hemlock (Conium maculatum), a lethal herbaceous perennial, thrives in damp, disturbed habitats

resembling those favored by wild carrot (Daucus carota), a non-toxic biennial with similar umbel-shaped flower clusters. Observing habitat preferences, soil conditions, and associated plant species aids in spatial awareness, risk assessment, and informed decision-making to avoid accidental ingestion of toxic plants mistaken for medicinal herbs.

Safety Precautions

Safety precautions in herbal medicine encompass proactive measures, risk assessment strategies, and contingency plans to minimize potential hazards associated with botanical preparations, toxic exposures, or adverse reactions. Herbalists prioritize client safety through comprehensive intake assessments, informed consent, and ongoing monitoring to ensure responsible use of herbal remedies tailored to individual health needs, preferences, and treatment goals.

1. **Education and Empowerment:** Education empowers individuals with essential knowledge, skills, and resources to make informed decisions about herbal use, plant identification, and safety precautions. Herbalists provide evidence-based information, practical guidance, and educational tools—such as botanical identification guides, toxic plant awareness seminars, and herbal safety workshops—to promote awareness, mitigate risks, and foster self-care practices rooted in botanical wisdom.

2. **Risk Assessment and Consultation:** Risk assessment involves systematic evaluation of potential hazards, contraindications, and adverse effects associated with herbal therapies, supporting informed decision-making and individualized treatment planning. Herbalists conduct thorough intake assessments, including medical history, allergies, concurrent medications, and lifestyle factors, to identify contraindications, mitigate risks, and tailor herbal formulations to optimize therapeutic outcomes safely. Collaboration with healthcare providers, toxicologists, and poison control centers facilitates timely intervention, multidisciplinary care, and emergency response protocols in managing herbal-related toxicities or adverse reactions effectively.

3. **Quality Assurance and Ethical Standards:** Quality assurance measures ensure integrity, purity, and safety in herbal preparations, emphasizing sustainable sourcing, organic cultivation practices, and rigorous quality control standards to minimize contaminants, adulterants, or variability in botanical constituents. Herbalists adhere to ethical principles, professional guidelines, and regulatory standards—such as Good Manufacturing Practices (GMP)—to uphold product integrity, consumer trust, and public safety in herbal medicine practice. Transparent labeling, dosage recommendations, and storage guidelines promote responsible use, informed decision-making, and optimal health outcomes for individuals and communities worldwide.

Identifying toxic look-alikes and implementing safety precautions are integral to safe and effective herbal medicine practice, fostering trust, confidence, and ethical stewardship in botanical therapies. By enhancing botanical proficiency, risk assessment strategies, and client education, herbalists promote informed decision-making, mitigate potential risks, and uphold patient safety throughout the therapeutic journey. Through collaboration, continuous learning, and shared responsibility, we advance the integration of herbal medicine within comprehensive healthcare frameworks, advocating for sustainable practices, cultural diversity, and holistic wellness in safeguarding the future of herbalism for generations to come.

5

Cultivation and Harvesting

Cultivation and harvesting play pivotal roles in the practice of herbal medicine, bridging botanical wisdom with sustainable practices to cultivate, harvest, and steward nature's pharmacy for therapeutic use. Herbalists embrace a holistic approach to plant cultivation, integrating ecological stewardship, seasonal rhythms, and traditional knowledge to cultivate medicinal herbs with potency, purity, and therapeutic efficacy. Through mindful cultivation practices and ethical harvesting techniques, herbalists honor the interconnectedness of plant health, environmental sustainability, and human well-being, fostering a symbiotic relationship between medicinal plants and holistic health.

In the chapters that follow, we explore the art and science of cultivating medicinal herbs—from seed to harvest—emphasizing soil health, biodiversity conservation, and regenerative agriculture practices that promote optimal plant growth, vitality, and medicinal potency. By nurturing herbal gardens, wildcrafting responsibly, and supporting community-based initiatives, herbalists nurture a legacy of botanical diversity, cultural resilience, and healing traditions that transcend generations. As guardians of nature's pharmacy, we celebrate the transformative potential of herbs as allies in promoting vitality, resilience, and sustainable wellness for individuals and communities worldwide.

Growing Herbal Plants in Different Environments

Growing herbal plants in diverse environments embraces the adaptability and resilience of botanical species to thrive in varying climates, soil conditions, and ecological niches. Herbalists leverage ecological knowledge, climate data, and site-specific considerations to cultivate medicinal herbs effectively, harnessing nature's diversity to optimize plant health, vitality, and therapeutic potency. From temperate gardens to arid landscapes, coastal habitats to mountainous regions, adapting cultivation practices ensures sustainable herbal production, ecological stewardship, and cultural relevance in herbal medicine practice.

1. Climate Considerations: Climate influences plant growth cycles, phenological events, and physiological responses that shape herbal medicine production in different environments. Mediterranean herbs—such as rosemary (Rosmarinus officinalis), lavender (Lavandula spp.), and thyme (Thymus spp.)—thrive in warm, dry climates with well-drained soils, benefiting from ample

sunlight and minimal moisture to enhance essential oil production and aromatic potency. Temperate herbs—like chamomile (Matricaria chamomilla), lemon balm (Melissa officinalis), and echinacea (Echinacea spp.)—adapt to moderate temperatures, regular rainfall, and fertile soils, supporting robust growth, floral abundance, and medicinal efficacy throughout the growing season.

2. **Soil Health and Fertility:** Soil health and fertility serve as foundational elements for cultivating healthy, nutrient-rich herbs that optimize medicinal potency and therapeutic benefits. Herbalists prioritize organic soil amendments, composting practices, and soil testing to assess nutrient levels, pH balance, and microbial diversity essential for plant growth, root development, and nutrient uptake. Well-drained soils, enriched with organic matter, support microbial symbiosis, water retention, and nutrient cycling, fostering resilient herbal gardens capable of sustaining diverse species and promoting long-term soil health in agricultural landscapes.

Best Practices for Harvesting

Best practices for harvesting herbal plants emphasize ecological ethics, seasonal rhythms, and plant-specific techniques to preserve medicinal potency, minimize environmental impact, and promote sustainable harvests. Herbalists integrate botanical knowledge, harvesting guidelines, and traditional wisdom to gather herbs at peak potency, honoring plant resilience, and ensuring quality assurance throughout the harvesting process.

1. **Timing and Phenological Indicators:** Timing of harvest aligns with phenological indicators—such as flowering stages, leaf maturity, and seed development—that signal optimal biochemical composition and medicinal efficacy in herbal plants. Harvesting flowers at full bloom—like calendula (Calendula officinalis) or elderflower (Sambucus nigra)—maximizes volatile oil content, flavonoid concentrations, and antioxidant properties essential for herbal infusions, tinctures, and skincare formulations. Leafy herbs—such as nettle (Urtica dioica) or peppermint (Mentha × piperita)—are

harvested before flowering to preserve leaf quality, essential oil yields, and bioactive compounds central to digestive health, respiratory support, and stress reduction.

2. **Ethical Wildcrafting Practices:** Ethical wildcrafting honors sustainable harvesting practices, cultural traditions, and ecological integrity in gathering wild medicinal plants from natural habitats, forests, or wild landscapes. Herbalists prioritize stewardship, conservation, and responsible harvesting permits to protect endangered species, fragile ecosystems, and biodiversity hotspots threatened by habitat loss or overexploitation. Wildcrafters collaborate with indigenous communities, conservation organizations, and land managers to promote ethical sourcing, ecological restoration, and community-based initiatives that sustainably manage wild medicinal plant populations for future generations.

3. **Post-Harvest Handling and Processing:** Post-harvest handling involves immediate processing, drying, or preservation techniques to maintain herb quality, potency, and shelf life essential for herbal medicine production. Herbalists employ gentle harvesting methods, shade drying, or low-temperature drying facilities to prevent heat degradation, moisture retention, or fungal contamination that compromise herb integrity and therapeutic efficacy. Proper storage conditions—such as cool, dark, and well-ventilated spaces—protect dried herbs from light exposure, oxidation, and moisture fluctuations, ensuring optimal storage stability and herbal quality for culinary, medicinal, and cosmetic applications.

Growing herbal plants in diverse environments and practicing best harvesting techniques embody the artistry and responsibility of herbal medicine, fostering ecological stewardship, cultural resilience, and sustainable wellness for individuals and communities worldwide. By adapting cultivation practices to environmental factors, embracing seasonal rhythms, and honoring plant wisdom through ethical harvesting, herbalists cultivate resilience, biodiversity, and therapeutic efficacy in medicinal herbs that nurture holistic health and promote planetary well-being. Through shared knowledge, collaborative partnerships, and lifelong learning, we celebrate the transformative potential of herbs as allies in promoting vitality, resilience, and sustainable wellness across generations, ensuring a future where botanical diversity thrives and healing flourishes for all.

Storing Herbal Plants

Proper storage of herbal plants is crucial to maintaining their medicinal potency, freshness, and therapeutic efficacy. After meticulous cultivation and thoughtful harvesting, the next critical step in herbal medicine practice is ensuring that these precious plants retain their beneficial properties until they are ready to be used. Effective storage techniques protect herbs from environmental factors that can degrade their quality, such as light, moisture, air, and temperature fluctuations.

1. Drying Methods: Drying is a fundamental method for preserving herbs. The process reduces the moisture content in plant material, preventing mold growth and decomposition while concentrating active compounds. Herbalists employ various drying techniques, such as air drying, dehydrating, or using drying racks and screens in well-ventilated, shaded areas. The key is to maintain low, steady temperatures and good airflow to ensure even drying without compromising the herbs' natural oils and constituents.

2. Storage Containers and Conditions: Once dried, herbs should be stored in airtight containers to protect them from exposure to air and moisture, which can cause oxidation and spoilage. Glass jars with tight-fitting lids, opaque containers, or vacuum-sealed bags are ideal for maintaining the freshness and potency of dried herbs. Herbalists often store herbs in dark, cool, and dry locations, away from direct sunlight and humidity, to further preserve their therapeutic properties. Labeling containers with the plant name, harvest date, and storage instructions ensures proper usage and rotation of stock.

3. Long-Term Storage Solutions: For herbs that need to be stored for extended periods, freezing or refrigeration can be effective. Freezing herbs like basil (Ocimum basilicum) or mint (Mentha spp.) in small, airtight containers or ice cube trays preserves their volatile oils and flavor, making them readily available for culinary and medicinal use. Refrigeration of fresh herbs like ginger (Zingiber officinale) or turmeric (Curcuma longa)

extends their shelf life and prevents spoilage, ensuring they remain potent and ready for use when needed.

Sustainable and Ethical Wildcrafting Methods

Sustainable and ethical wildcrafting embodies a profound respect for nature, cultural traditions, and ecological integrity. Wildcrafting, or the practice of harvesting plants from their natural habitats, requires a deep understanding of plant ecology, conservation principles, and ethical guidelines to ensure that wild plant populations thrive for future generations.

1. Conservation and Biodiversity: Sustainable wildcrafting prioritizes the conservation of plant species and their habitats, ensuring that harvesting practices do not threaten the survival of wild populations or disrupt local ecosystems. Herbalists conduct thorough assessments of plant populations, growth cycles, and ecological roles before harvesting, taking care to leave enough plants to reproduce and maintain ecological balance. Harvesting only a small percentage of the available plant material, avoiding rare or endangered species, and practicing rotational harvesting are essential strategies for preserving biodiversity and ecological health.

2. Ethical Harvesting Techniques: Ethical wildcrafting involves respectful and mindful harvesting techniques that minimize harm to plants and their environments. Herbalists use tools that cause minimal damage, such as sharp knives or scissors, and avoid uprooting entire plants unless necessary for specific roots or rhizomes. Harvesting during optimal times—when plants are most potent and resilient—ensures minimal impact on their growth and regeneration. Additionally, herbalists practice gratitude and reciprocity, acknowledging the gifts of nature and giving back through seed scattering, habitat restoration, and community education.

3. Community and Cultural Respect: Wildcrafting is deeply rooted in cultural traditions and indigenous knowledge systems. Herbalists honor the wisdom and practices of indigenous communities by seeking permission, collaborating, and adhering to local guidelines and customs. Building relationships with

indigenous stewards of the land fosters mutual respect, knowledge exchange, and cultural preservation. Herbalists advocate for equitable access to wildcrafting sites, fair compensation for indigenous contributions, and the protection of sacred or culturally significant plants.

Storing herbal plants and practicing sustainable and ethical wildcrafting methods are integral to the integrity and efficacy of herbal medicine. By employing meticulous storage techniques, herbalists preserve the potency, freshness, and therapeutic properties of herbs, ensuring their availability for healing and well-being. Through sustainable and ethical wildcrafting, we honor the interconnectedness of plant health, ecological stewardship, and cultural respect, fostering a harmonious relationship with nature that nurtures biodiversity, resilience, and sustainable wellness for all.

6

Recipes and Applications

Herbal medicine is a timeless tradition that bridges ancient wisdom with modern wellness practices, utilizing the remarkable properties of plants to promote health, prevent illness, and enhance overall well-being. Central to this practice is the art of transforming raw botanical materials into accessible, effective remedies through a variety of recipes and applications. Whether through soothing teas, invigorating tinctures, nourishing salves, or aromatic infusions, these preparations harness the therapeutic potential of herbs in ways that are both practical and profoundly healing.

In this chapter, we delve into the diverse world of herbal recipes and applications, exploring how different methods of preparation can unlock the medicinal virtues of plants and make them readily available for everyday use. Each method offers unique benefits and serves specific purposes, tailored to address various health needs and preferences. By understanding the principles behind these preparations, you can confidently incorporate herbs into your daily routine, creating personalized remedies that support your journey towards optimal health.

Herbal Remedies: Step-by-Step Instructions

Herbal remedies offer a natural and holistic approach to health and wellness, drawing on centuries of traditional knowledge and the therapeutic properties of plants. By following detailed, step-by-step instructions, you can create a variety of herbal preparations tailored to your specific needs, from soothing teas to potent tinctures and nourishing salves. In this section, we will explore these methods in depth, empowering you to incorporate herbal medicine into your daily life with confidence and passion.

Herbal Teas

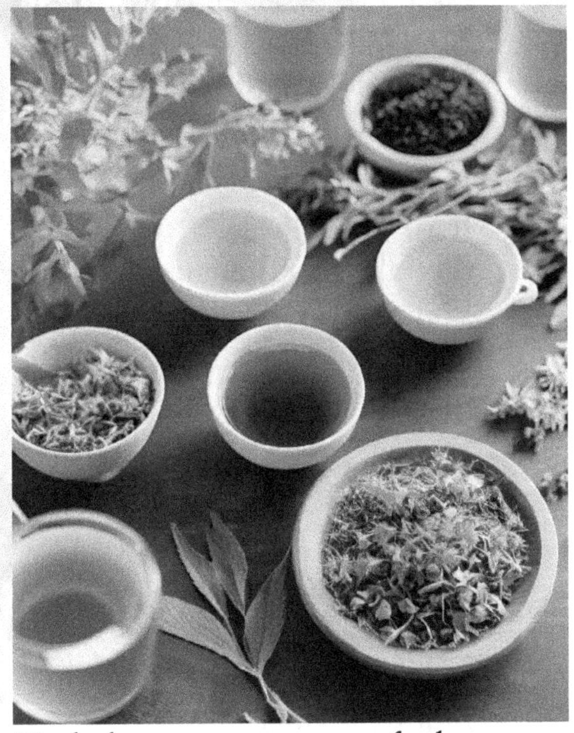

Herbal teas are one of the most accessible forms of herbal medicine.

They are easy to prepare, gentle on the body, and can be enjoyed daily to support overall health and well-being.

Step-by-Step Instructions for Making Herbal Teas:

1. **Select Your Herbs:** Choose herbs based on their medicinal properties and your specific needs. For example, chamomile (Matricaria chamomilla) for relaxation, peppermint (Mentha × piperita) for digestion, or elderberry (Sambucus nigra) for immune support.
2. **Measure the Herbs:** Use approximately 1-2 teaspoons of dried herbs or 2-3 teaspoons of fresh herbs per cup of water. Adjust the quantity based on the desired strength of the tea.
3. **Boil the Water:** Bring fresh, filtered water to a boil. The quality of the water can affect the taste and efficacy of the tea.
4. **Infuse the Herbs:** Place the herbs in a teapot, infuser, or directly into the cup. Pour the boiling water over the herbs and cover to prevent the volatile oils from escaping.
5. **Steep the Tea:** Allow the herbs to steep for 5-10 minutes, depending on the type of herb and desired strength. Delicate herbs like flowers may need less time, while roots and barks may require a longer steep.
6. **Strain and Enjoy:** Strain the herbs from the tea using a fine mesh strainer or tea infuser. Pour the tea into your cup, sweeten with honey or lemon if desired, and enjoy the soothing effects.

Tinctures

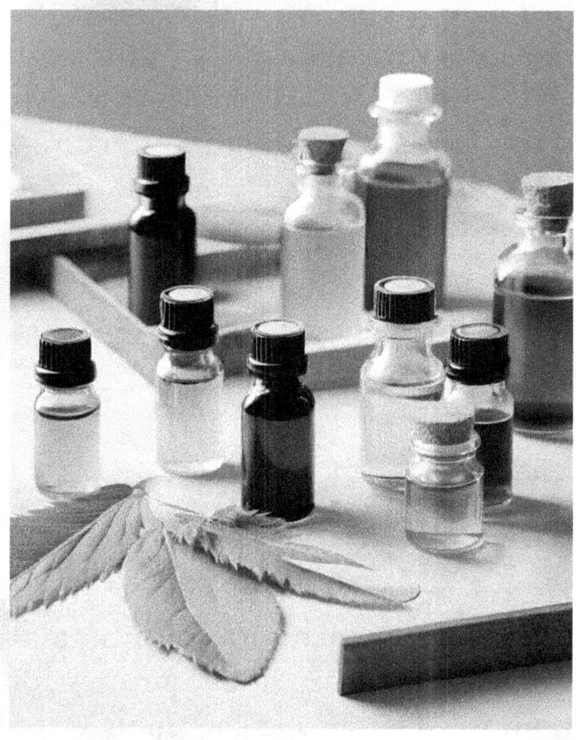

Tinctures are alcohol-based extracts that provide a potent and convenient way to consume herbal medicine. They are especially useful for those seeking strong, fast-acting relief.

Step-by-Step Instructions for Making Tinctures:

1. **Choose Your Herbs:** Select fresh or dried herbs based on their therapeutic properties. Common choices include echinacea (Echinacea spp.) for immune support, valerian (Valeriana officinalis) for sleep,

and milk thistle (**Silybum marianum**) **for liver health.**

2. **Prepare the Herbs:** Chop fresh herbs finely or crush dried herbs to increase the surface area for extraction. Measure the herbs by weight to ensure consistent potency.

3. **Select the Solvent:** Use a high-proof alcohol (such as vodka or brandy) for fresh herbs or a lower-proof alcohol (40-60%) for dried herbs. Alcohol extracts a wide range of plant constituents, ensuring a potent tincture.

4. **Combine Herbs and Alcohol:** Place the herbs in a clean glass jar and cover with alcohol, ensuring the herbs are fully submerged. The ratio of herbs to alcohol is typically 1:2 for fresh herbs and 1:5 for dried herbs.

5. **Seal and Shake:** Seal the jar tightly and shake well to mix. Store the jar in a cool, dark place, shaking it daily to enhance extraction.

6. **Steep for Several Weeks:** Allow the mixture to steep for 4-6 weeks, giving the alcohol time to extract the medicinal compounds from the herbs.

7. **Strain and Bottle:** After the steeping period, strain the mixture through a fine mesh strainer or cheesecloth, squeezing out as much liquid as possible. Transfer the tincture to dark glass bottles and label with the herb name, alcohol type, and date.

8. **Dosage and Use:** Use tinctures as directed, typically 1-2 dropperfuls (approximately 30-60 drops) diluted in water, juice, or directly under the tongue. Consult a herbalist for personalized dosing guidelines.

Salves and Balms

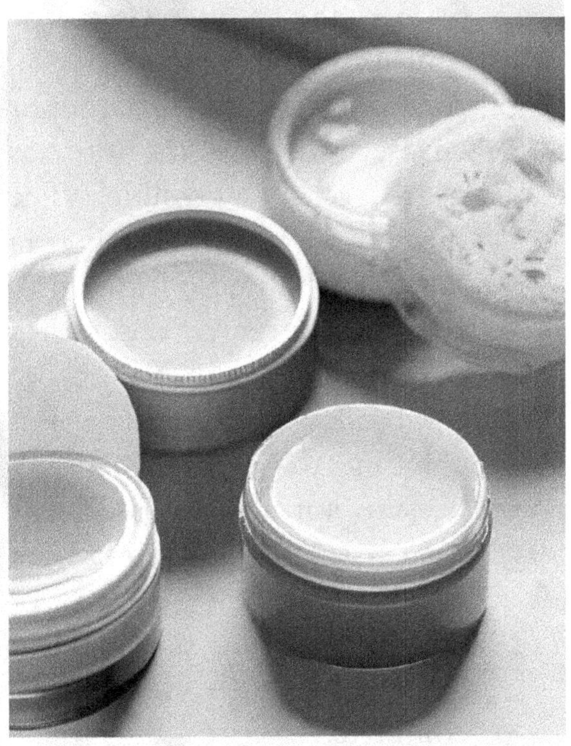

Salves and balms are thick, oil-based preparations infused with healing herbs, ideal for soothing skin conditions, muscle pain, and minor wounds.

Step-by-Step Instructions for Making Salves:

1. **Select Your Herbs and Oils:** Choose herbs with skin-healing properties, such as calendula (Calendula officinalis), comfrey

(Symphytum officinale), and plantain (Plantago major). Select a carrier oil like olive oil, coconut oil, or almond oil.

2. **Infuse the Oil:** Combine the herbs and carrier oil in a clean, dry glass jar. Use a ratio of 1 part dried herbs to 2-3 parts oil. Seal the jar and place it in a sunny windowsill or warm spot, shaking it daily. Allow the herbs to infuse for 4-6 weeks.

3. **Strain the Oil:** After the infusion period, strain the oil through a fine mesh strainer or cheesecloth, pressing out as much oil as possible. The infused oil can be stored in a dark glass bottle for future use.

4. **Prepare the Salve Base:** In a double boiler or heatproof bowl set over simmering water, combine the infused oil with beeswax (or a plant-based wax for a vegan option) in a ratio of approximately 1 ounce of beeswax per cup of oil. Heat gently until the wax melts completely.

5. **Add Essential Oils:** If desired, add a few drops of essential oils for additional therapeutic benefits and fragrance. Lavender (Lavandula angustifolia) and tea tree (Melaleuca alternifolia) oils are popular choices for skin-healing salves.

6. **Pour into Containers:** Pour the melted mixture into clean, dry tins or glass jars. Allow the salve to cool and solidify completely before sealing the containers.

7. **Label and Store:** Label the containers with the ingredients and date. Store the salves in a cool, dark place to extend their shelf life. They can typically be used for up to one year.

8. **Application:** Apply the salve to the affected area as needed, massaging gently to aid absorption. Use for dry skin, minor cuts and scrapes, insect bites, and muscle aches.

Infusions and Decoctions

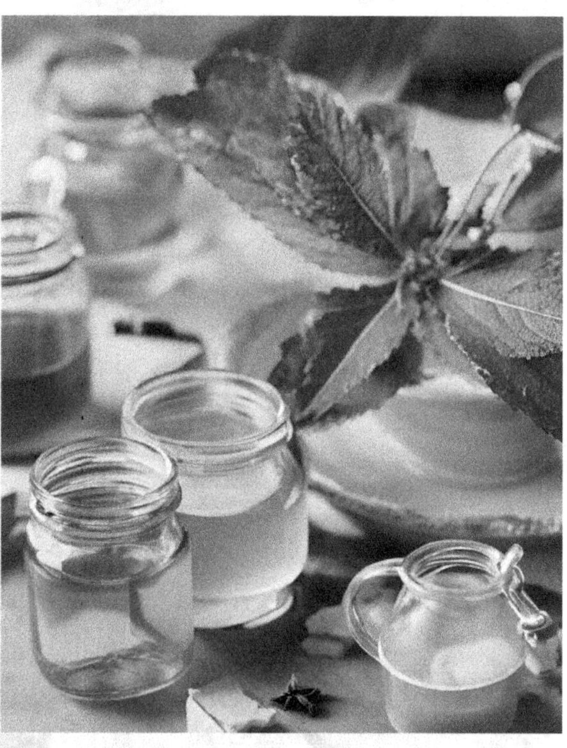

Infusions and decoctions are methods of extracting the medicinal compounds of herbs through prolonged steeping or simmering in water.

Step-by-Step Instructions for Making Infusions:

1. Select Your Herbs: Choose herbs suited for infusions, such as nettle (Urtica dioica) for mineral content, oat straw (Avena sativa) for nervous system support, or red clover (Trifolium pratense) for hormonal balance.
2. Measure the Herbs: Use approximately 1 ounce of dried herbs per quart of water for a nourishing infusion. Adjust the quantity based on the desired strength.
3. Boil the Water: Bring fresh, filtered water to a rolling boil.
4. Steep the Herbs: Place the herbs in a heatproof jar or French press. Pour the boiling water over the herbs, cover, and let steep for 4-8 hours or overnight to extract the maximum amount of nutrients and medicinal compounds.
5. Strain and Store: Strain the infusion through a fine mesh strainer or cheesecloth. Store the liquid in a clean, sealed container in the refrigerator for up to 3 days.
6. Dosage and Use: Drink 1-3 cups of the infusion daily, cold or gently warmed. Infusions can also be used in baths or as a base for other herbal preparations.

Step-by-Step Instructions for Making Decoctions:

1. Select Your Herbs: Choose tougher plant materials like roots, barks, and seeds for decoctions. Common choices include ginger root (Zingiber officinale) for digestion, licorice root (Glycyrrhiza glabra) for respiratory support, and cinnamon bark (Cinnamomum verum) for blood sugar balance.
2. Measure the Herbs: Use approximately 1 ounce of dried herbs per quart of water for a decoction.
3. Combine Herbs and Water: Place the herbs and water in a heavy-bottomed pot.
4. Simmer the Decoction: Bring the mixture to a boil, then reduce the heat and let it simmer gently for 20-30 minutes. For very tough roots or barks, simmer for up to an hour.
5. Cool and Strain: Remove from heat and allow the decoction to cool slightly. Strain the liquid through a fine mesh strainer or cheesecloth.
6. Store and Use: Store the decoction in a clean, sealed container in the refrigerator for up to 3 days. Drink 1-3 cups daily, or use as directed for specific health conditions.

Culinary Applications

Integrating medicinal herbs into your cooking allows you to enjoy their health benefits in a delicious and natural way.

Step-by-Step Instructions for Culinary Applications:

Herb-Infused Oils and Vinegars:

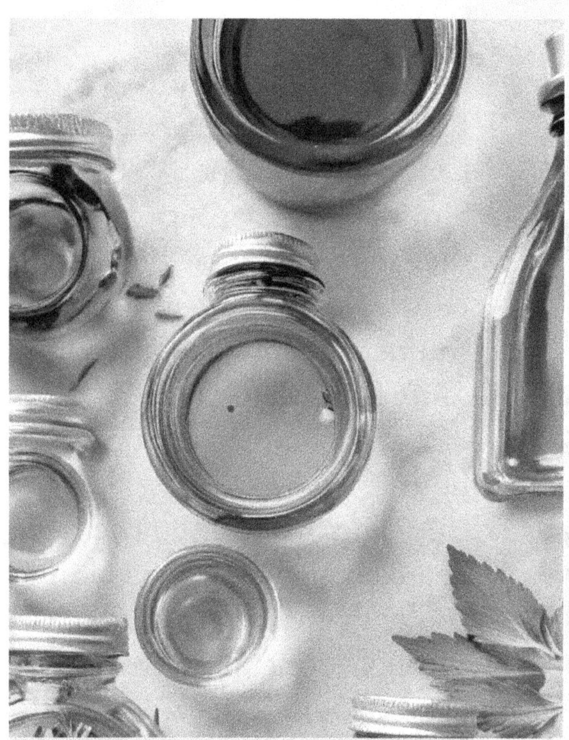

1. Select Your Herbs: Choose aromatic herbs like rosemary (Rosmarinus officinalis), thyme (Thymus spp.), or basil (Ocimum basilicum).
2. Prepare the Herbs: Wash and dry the herbs thoroughly. Slightly bruise them to release their oils.
3. Combine with Oil or Vinegar: Place the herbs in a clean, dry glass bottle. Fill the bottle with your choice of olive oil, vinegar, or another preferred base, ensuring the herbs are fully submerged.
4. Infuse the Mixture: Seal the bottle tightly and store it in a cool, dark place. Allow the mixture to infuse for 2-4 weeks, shaking it gently every few days.
5. Strain and Use: Strain the herbs out of the oil or vinegar and transfer the infused liquid to a clean bottle. Label the bottle with the contents and date. Use the herb-infused oil or vinegar to dress salads, marinate meats, or enhance the flavor of your favorite dishes.

Herbal Butters:

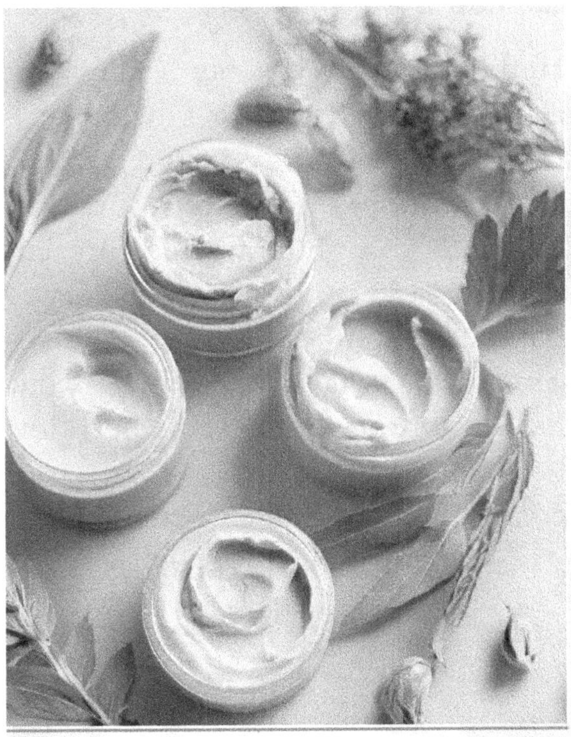

1. **Select Your Herbs:** Choose fresh herbs like parsley (Petroselinum crispum), dill (Anethum graveolens), or chives (Allium schoenoprasum).
2. **Prepare the Butter:** Soften a stick of unsalted butter at room temperature.
3. **Chop the Herbs:** Finely chop the fresh herbs and mix them into the softened butter. Add a pinch of salt and any other seasonings you like.
4. **Shape and Chill:** Transfer the herb butter to a piece of parchment paper. Roll it into a log shape, twisting the ends of the paper to seal. Chill the herb butter in the refrigerator until firm.
5. **Use and Enjoy:** Slice the herb butter as needed to spread on bread, melt over vegetables, or use to flavor cooked meats and fish.

Herbal Honey:

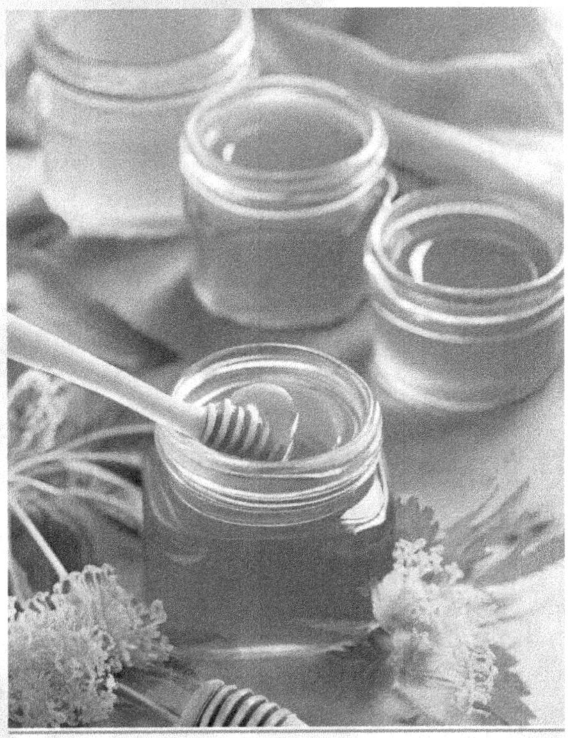

1. **Select Your Herbs:** Choose aromatic herbs like lavender (Lavandula angustifolia), chamomile (Matricaria chamomilla), or lemon balm (Melissa officinalis).
2. **Combine with Honey:** Place the herbs in a clean, dry glass jar. Pour raw honey over the herbs until they are fully submerged.
3. **Infuse the Honey:** Seal the jar and let the mixture infuse in a warm, sunny spot for 1-2 weeks, stirring occasionally.
4. **Strain and Use:** Strain the herbs out of the honey and transfer the infused honey to a

clean jar. Use it to sweeten tea, drizzle over yogurt, or add to your favorite recipes.

Herbal remedies offer a versatile and natural way to support health and well-being. By following these step-by-step instructions, you can create a variety of herbal preparations tailored to your needs, from soothing teas and potent tinctures to nourishing salves and flavorful culinary creations. Each method allows you to harness the therapeutic properties of herbs in unique and effective ways, enriching your daily life with the healing power of nature.

Herbs have been our allies for centuries, offering their gifts to heal, nourish, and inspire. By incorporating them into your daily routine, you honor this ancient tradition and contribute to a legacy of natural wellness that spans generations. As you continue your herbal journey, may you find joy, healing, and a profound sense of connection with the natural world.

Household Applications

Herbs are not only valuable for their culinary, medicinal, and cosmetic uses but also offer numerous benefits for the household. Integrating herbs into your daily home care routines can transform your living space into a haven of natural wellness and aromatic pleasure. Below, we explore various household applications of herbs, from natural cleaning solutions to pest repellents and aromatic enhancers.

Natural Cleaning Solutions

Herbs can be powerful allies in keeping your home clean and fresh without relying on harsh chemicals. Their natural antibacterial, antifungal, and antiseptic properties make them ideal for creating effective and pleasant-smelling cleaning products.

Step-by-Step Instructions for Herbal Cleaning Solutions:

Herbal All-Purpose Cleaner:

1. Select Your Herbs: Choose herbs like lavender (Lavandula angustifolia), thyme (Thymus spp.), and rosemary (Rosmarinus officinalis) for their antimicrobial properties.
2. Prepare an Infusion: Boil water and pour it over the fresh or dried herbs. Let the herbs steep until the water cools to room temperature.
3. Combine with Vinegar: Strain the herbal infusion and mix it with equal parts white vinegar in a spray bottle.

4. Add Essential Oils: For an extra boost of fragrance and cleaning power, add a few drops of essential oils like tea tree (Melaleuca alternifolia) or lemon (Citrus limon).
5. Use for Cleaning: Shake well before use. Spray the mixture on countertops, sinks, and other surfaces, then wipe clean with a cloth.

Herbal Floor Cleaner:

1. Select Your Herbs: Eucalyptus (Eucalyptus globulus) and peppermint (Mentha piperita) are excellent choices for their refreshing scent and cleaning properties.
2. Prepare an Infusion: Steep the herbs in boiling water until it cools.
3. Combine with Castile Soap: Strain the infusion and mix it with a few tablespoons of liquid Castile soap.
4. Mop Your Floors: Add the mixture to a bucket of warm water and use it to mop your floors, leaving them clean and fragrant.

Herbal Air Fresheners:

1. Select Your Herbs: Use aromatic herbs like basil (Ocimum basilicum), mint (Mentha spp.), and sage (Salvia officinalis).
2. Prepare a Simmer Pot: Add the herbs to a pot of water and bring it to a gentle simmer. The steam will release their fragrant oils into the air, naturally freshening your home.
3. Essential Oil Spray: Alternatively, mix a few drops of essential oils with water in a spray bottle. Use this to spritz your home for a quick and easy air freshener.

Herbal Pest Repellents

Herbs can help keep your home free from pests without resorting to synthetic chemicals. Their natural repellent properties can deter insects and rodents, creating a healthier living environment.

Step-by-Step Instructions for Herbal Pest Repellents:

Herbal Insect Repellent:

1. Select Your Herbs: Use herbs like citronella (Cymbopogon nardus), lemongrass (Cymbopogon citratus), and lavender (Lavandula angustifolia).
2. Prepare an Infusion: Steep the herbs in boiling water and allow them to cool.
3. Combine with Witch Hazel: Strain the infusion and mix it with equal parts witch hazel in a spray bottle.

4. Add Essential Oils: Enhance the repellent effect by adding a few drops of essential oils like eucalyptus (Eucalyptus globulus) and peppermint (Mentha piperita).
5. Spray and Protect: Use the mixture to spray around doorways, windows, and other entry points to keep insects at bay.

Herbal Rodent Repellent:

1. Select Your Herbs: Peppermint (Mentha piperita) and spearmint (Mentha spicata) are effective for deterring rodents.
2. Prepare Herbal Sachets: Fill small cloth bags with dried peppermint and spearmint leaves.
3. Place Strategically: Place the sachets in areas where rodents are likely to enter, such as cabinets, pantries, and corners.
4. Refresh Regularly: Replace the herbs periodically to maintain their effectiveness.

Aromatic Enhancers

Herbs can also be used to enhance the atmosphere of your home with their pleasant and calming scents. From potpourri to herbal candles, these aromatic enhancers create a soothing and inviting environment.

Step-by-Step Instructions for Aromatic Enhancers:

Herbal Potpourri:

1. Select Your Herbs: Choose a variety of fragrant herbs and flowers, such as rose petals (Rosa spp.), lavender (Lavandula angustifolia), and lemon balm (Melissa officinalis).
2. Prepare and Dry the Herbs: Collect and dry the herbs and flowers until they are completely moisture-free.
3. Mix and Store: Combine the dried herbs and flowers in a decorative bowl or jar. Add a few drops of essential oils for added fragrance.
4. Refresh the Scent: Stir the potpourri occasionally and add more essential oils as needed to maintain the scent.

Herbal Candles:

1. Select Your Herbs: Use dried herbs like rosemary (Rosmarinus officinalis), sage (Salvia officinalis), and chamomile (Matricaria chamomilla).
2. Prepare the Candle Wax: Melt natural beeswax or soy wax in a double boiler.

3. **Add Herbs and Essential Oils:** Stir in the dried herbs and a few drops of essential oils.

4. **Pour into Molds:** Pour the wax mixture into candle molds, ensuring the wick is centered.

5. **Cool and Set:** Allow the candles to cool and set completely before removing them from the molds.

6. **Use for Ambiance:** Light the herbal candles to enjoy their soothing aroma and natural ambiance.

Herbal Sachets for Closets and Drawers:

1. **Select Your Herbs:** Lavender (Lavandula angustifolia), cedar (Cedrus spp.), and rosemary (Rosmarinus officinalis) are great choices for keeping clothes and linens fresh.

2. **Prepare the Sachets:** Fill small cloth bags with dried herbs and tie them securely.

3. **Place in Storage Areas:** Place the sachets in closets, drawers, and storage boxes to infuse your fabrics with a pleasant herbal scent and deter moths and other pests.

4. **Refresh Regularly:** Replace or replenish the herbs as their scent fades.

Incorporating herbs into your household routines not only enhances the aesthetic and sensory appeal of your home but also promotes a healthier, more natural living environment. From natural cleaning solutions and pest repellents to aromatic enhancers, herbs offer a versatile and effective way to maintain your home.

7

Key Botanical Features for Identification

As herbalists, our ability to accurately identify plants lies at the heart of our practice. Understanding the key botanical features of plants allows us to confidently distinguish between species, assess their medicinal properties, and ensure their safe and effective use. This chapter delves into the essential characteristics that define plant species, offering a detailed exploration of their morphology, structures, and distinctive traits. By mastering these botanical features, we empower ourselves to navigate the rich diversity of herbal flora with precision and expertise, furthering our commitment to harnessing nature's healing bounty responsibly and effectively.

Leaf Shapes and Arrangements

Leaves are the primary organs of photosynthesis and serve as key identifiers in plant taxonomy. Their shapes and arrangements exhibit a stunning diversity, each adaptation finely tuned to the plant's ecological niche and evolutionary history. By understanding these characteristics, herbalists gain insights into a plant's identity, medicinal potential, and environmental adaptations.

Leaf Shapes:

- Simple Leaves: These are single, undivided leaves that may vary widely in shape. Examples include the oval leaves of basil (Ocimum basilicum), the lance-shaped leaves of plantain (Plantago spp.), and the heart-shaped leaves of violet (Viola spp.). Each shape reflects adaptations to light exposure, water availability, and nutrient uptake strategies.

- Compound Leaves: Compound leaves consist of leaflets arranged along a central stalk or rachis. This arrangement enhances flexibility and light capture. Examples include the trifoliate leaves of clover (Trifolium spp.) and the pinnate leaves of neem (Azadirachta indica). The complexity of compound leaves offers clues to a plant's evolutionary relationships and ecological functions.

- Needle-like Leaves: Found in conifers such as pine (Pinus spp.) and juniper (Juniperus spp.), needle-like leaves are adapted for reduced water loss in arid environments. Their slender shape minimizes surface area exposed to drying winds, while specialized stomata and thick cuticles further conserve water.

- Scale-like Leaves: Scale-like leaves are characteristic of plants like cypress (Cupressus spp.) and cedar (Cedrus spp.). These flattened structures overlap tightly, reducing water loss and protecting against herbivory in harsh climates. Their arrangement reflects adaptations to cold or dry conditions, emphasizing resilience over rapid growth.

Leaf Arrangements:

- **Alternate Arrangement:** In alternate leaf arrangement, leaves emerge singly along the stem, alternating sides with each node. This pattern allows for efficient light capture and minimizes shading among leaves. Examples include the leaves of rose (Rosa spp.) and sunflower (Helianthus annuus), which maximize exposure to sunlight.

- **Opposite Arrangement:** Leaves in opposite arrangement grow in pairs at each node, directly opposite each other. This symmetrical pattern is seen in plants like mint (Mentha spp.) and lilac (Syringa vulgaris). Opposite leaves often indicate specific adaptations for efficient nutrient uptake or mechanical support in vertical growth.

- **Whorled Arrangement:** Whorled leaves radiate from multiple points around the stem, forming a circle or spiral. This arrangement is less common but seen in plants like Galium spp. (bedstraw) and Asclepias spp. (milkweed). Whorled leaves may optimize light capture in crowded environments or reflect adaptations to specialized habitats.

Flower Structures and Types

Flowers represent the reproductive pinnacle of plants, showcasing a remarkable array of structures, colors, and scents to attract pollinators and ensure species survival. From the delicate symmetry of petals to the intricate arrangements of reproductive organs, understanding flower structures enriches our appreciation of plant diversity and their roles in ecosystems.

Flower Structures:

- **Petal Arrangement:** Petals form the colorful outer whorl of the flower, attracting pollinators with hues ranging from vibrant reds to subtle pastels. They may be fused or separate, forming tubular, bell-shaped, or flat structures. Examples include the fused petals of a morning glory

(Ipomoea spp.) or the separate petals of a daisy (Bellis perennis).

- **Sepal Shapes:** Sepals protect the developing flower bud and often resemble modified leaves. They may be green, resembling leaves, or brightly colored, enhancing floral display. Sepals can be fused or separate, forming a protective covering that opens as the flower blooms. Variations in sepal shape and texture provide clues to a flower's ecological adaptations.

- **Stamen and Pistil:** The stamen comprises the male reproductive organs, consisting of anthers (where pollen is produced) and filaments (supporting the anthers). The pistil is the female reproductive organ, consisting of the stigma (where pollen lands), style (connecting stigma to ovary), and ovary (containing ovules). The arrangement and size of stamens and pistils vary widely among species, influencing pollination mechanisms and seed development.

Flower Types:

- **Actinomorphic Flowers:** Actinomorphic flowers are radially symmetrical, with multiple planes of symmetry passing through the center. They are typical of plants pollinated by generalist insects, such as bees and butterflies. Examples include the flowers of roses (Rosa spp.) and buttercups (Ranunculus spp.), which attract pollinators with open, accessible nectar and pollen.

- **Zygomorphic Flowers:** Zygomorphic flowers exhibit bilateral symmetry, with only one plane of symmetry dividing the flower into mirror-image halves. This adaptation often targets specific pollinators, ensuring precise pollen transfer. Examples include the orchid (Orchidaceae) family, where intricate structures guide insects to specialized nectar rewards and pollen deposits

- **Inflorescence Types:** Inflorescences are clusters of flowers arranged on a single stem, enhancing floral display and pollination efficiency. Types include spikes (elongated, unbranched inflorescences like in lupines), racemes (unbranched with stalked flowers like in snapdragons), and umbels (flat-topped clusters like in dill). Inflorescence types reflect plant strategies for maximizing reproductive success and attracting diverse pollinators.

This exploration of leaf shapes, arrangements, flower structures, and types highlights the intricate adaptations and ecological strategies of plants. Each feature offers a window into a plant's evolutionary history, ecological niche, and interactions within its habitat. For herbalists, mastering these botanical details enriches our ability to identify, understand, and utilize plants for their medicinal and ecological value, fostering a deeper connection with the natural world.

Stem and Root Characteristics

Stems and roots serve as the vital conduits and anchors of plants, embodying adaptations that reflect their ecological roles and survival strategies. From sturdy anchors beneath the soil to resilient structures reaching towards the sun, understanding these botanical features unveils the resilience and diversity of plant life.

Stem Characteristics:

- **Stem Types:** Plants exhibit a variety of stem types, each adapted to support growth and transport nutrients. Herbaceous stems, such as those found in basil (Ocimum basilicum), are soft and flexible, ideal for rapid growth and seasonal adaptation. Woody stems, seen in trees like oak (Quercus spp.), provide durable support and protection, enabling long-term growth and structural integrity.
- **Stem Structures:** Stem structures vary widely across species, influencing plant architecture and resource allocation. Rhizomes, found in plants like ginger (Zingiber officinale), are underground stems that store nutrients and enable vegetative reproduction. Stolons, seen in strawberries (Fragaria spp.), are horizontal stems that root at nodes, facilitating spread and survival
- **Stem Modifications:** Modified stems adapt to diverse environmental challenges, enhancing plant survival and reproduction. Thorns, as seen in roses (Rosa spp.) and citrus trees (Citrus spp.), deter herbivores and protect vulnerable tissues. Tendrils, found in peas (Pisum spp.) and grapes (Vitis spp.), enable climbing and enhance access to light and support.

Root Characteristics:

- **Root Types:** Roots serve essential functions, anchoring plants and absorbing water and nutrients from the soil. Taproots, like those in carrots (Daucus carota), penetrate deeply for water uptake and storage. Fibrous roots, seen in grasses (Poaceae), form dense networks close to the soil surface, maximizing nutrient acquisition and stability.

- Root Structures: Root structures vary in complexity and adaptation, reflecting plant strategies for resource acquisition and storage. Adventitious roots, as in corn (Zea mays), emerge from stems or leaves to enhance stability and nutrient uptake. Storage roots, such as those in sweet potatoes (Ipomoea batatas), store reserves for seasonal or reproductive needs.

- Root Modifications: Modified roots fulfill specialized functions, enhancing plant survival and ecological interactions. Pneumatophores, seen in mangroves (Rhizophora spp.), project above water surfaces to facilitate gas exchange in oxygen-poor environments. Contractile roots, as in bulbs like onions (Allium spp.), pull the plant deeper into the soil, protecting it from drought and temperature fluctuations.

Scent and Other Sensory Identifiers

The sensory qualities of plants extend beyond visual identification, encompassing a symphony of scents, textures, and tastes that evoke their ecological roles and medicinal potential. From aromatic oils that deter pests to bitter compounds that signal toxicity, these sensory identifiers enrich our understanding and appreciation of plant diversity.

Aromatic Profiles:

- Essential Oils: Plants produce essential oils, concentrated compounds that imbue them with distinct fragrances and medicinal properties. Lavender (Lavandula angustifolia) yields calming oils used in aromatherapy, while peppermint (Mentha piperita) provides invigorating oils for digestive relief. These aromatic signatures guide herbalists in plant identification and therapeutic application.

- Scent Families: Floral, herbal, citrus, and spicy scents are categorized into scent families that reveal plant relationships and ecological adaptations. Roses (Rosa spp.) emit floral notes that attract pollinators, whereas eucalyptus (Eucalyptus spp.) releases medicinal scents that deter pests and promote respiratory health.

- Sensory Defense Mechanisms: Plants deploy sensory defense mechanisms through bitter, pungent, or astringent compounds that deter herbivores and pathogens. Bitter alkaloids in coffee

(Coffea spp.) and quinine (Cinchona spp.) signal toxicity, protecting plants while shaping their cultural and medicinal roles.

Texture and Taste:

- **Leaf Textures:** Leaf textures range from velvety softness in lamb's ear (Stachys byzantina) to waxy resilience in holly (Ilex spp.), reflecting adaptations to moisture retention and herbivore deterrence.
- **Flavor Profiles:** Culinary and medicinal herbs boast diverse flavor profiles, from the peppery warmth of basil (Ocimum basilicum) to the cooling freshness of mint (Mentha spp.). These tastes guide herbalists in culinary applications and therapeutic formulations, enriching human interactions with plants.
- **Tactile Feedback:** Plant textures provide tactile feedback that informs our interactions and cultural uses. Aloe vera (Aloe spp.) offers soothing gel for skin care, while thorny stems in roses (Rosa spp.) discourage handling.

This exploration of stem and root characteristics, as well as sensory identifiers, illuminates the intricate adaptations and sensory tapestry of plants. Each feature offers a gateway to understanding plant resilience, ecological roles, and human interactions. For herbalists, mastering these botanical details fosters deeper connections with nature's diversity, enriching our practice and stewardship of plant resources.

Conclusion

Throughout this journey of herbal plant identification, we have ventured into the intricate world of botanical features, sensory identifiers, and ecological adaptations that define plants. From the delicate symmetry of flower petals to the resilient structures of stems and roots, each chapter has unveiled nature's exquisite craftsmanship and evolutionary strategies. As herbalists, our quest to understand and appreciate these elements goes beyond mere identification—it embodies a profound connection with the natural world and a commitment to harnessing its healing gifts responsibly.

In exploring leaf shapes and arrangements, flower structures and types, we have celebrated the diversity of plant life. Each botanical feature serves as a testament to adaptation and survival, reflecting millennia of evolutionary refinement. By mastering these characteristics, we empower ourselves to recognize plants not only by their physical traits but also by their ecological roles and potential benefits.

The exploration of scent and other sensory identifiers has enriched our understanding of plants as sensory beings. Aromatic oils, bitter compounds, and tactile textures offer clues to their medicinal properties and ecological interactions. These sensory cues guide us in plant identification, therapeutic applications, and sustainable harvesting practices, ensuring that our interactions with plants are rooted in respect and reciprocity.

From culinary uses and medicinal preparations to household applications and ecological stewardship, the knowledge gained from identifying plants transcends mere academic pursuit. It empowers us to integrate herbs into daily life, enhancing health and wellness while fostering a deeper appreciation for nature's bounty. Whether crafting herbal remedies, creating natural cleaning solutions, or cultivating plants in diverse environments, our expertise in plant identification serves as a foundation for sustainable living and holistic well-being.

As stewards of herbal knowledge, we bear a profound responsibility to protect and preserve plant diversity. By recognizing the ecological significance of each species and practicing ethical wildcrafting methods, we ensure that future generations can benefit from nature's abundance. Our commitment to sustainability extends beyond individual practices—it shapes global efforts to conserve biodiversity and mitigate environmental impacts.

As we conclude this exploration of herbal plant identification, let us embrace a future where human health is intertwined with the health of our planet. Let us continue to study, respect, and advocate for the protection of herbal resources, acknowledging their intrinsic value and cultural significance. Through collaboration, education, and advocacy, we can empower communities to cultivate resilience and well-being through herbal wisdom.

In closing, the study of herbal plant identification is not merely a scientific pursuit—it is a journey of discovery, connection, and reverence for the natural world. May our continued exploration of plants inspire curiosity, deepen our understanding of ecological interconnectedness, and nurture a sense of gratitude for the gifts that plants offer us each day.